ITI Treatment Guide
Volume 1

ITI
Treatment
Guide

Editors:
D. Buser, U. Belser, D. Wismeijer

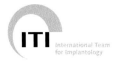
ITI International Team for Implantology

Authors:
U. Belser, W. Martin,
R. Jung, C. Hämmerle, B. Schmid,
D. Morton, D. Buser

Volume 1

Implant Therapy in the Esthetic Zone
Single-Tooth Replacements

Quintessence Publishing Co, Ltd
Berlin, Chicago, London, Tokyo, Barcelona,
Beijing, Istanbul, Milan, Moscow, Mumbai,
Paris, Prague, São Paulo, Seoul, Warsaw

German National Library CIP Data

The German National Library has listed this publication in the German National Bibliography. Detailed bibliographical data are available on the Internet at http://dnb.ddb.de.

 © 2007 Quintessence Publishing Co, Ltd
Ifenpfad 2-4, 12107 Berlin,
www.quintessenz.de

Medical Editing: Dr. Kati Benthaus, CH-Basel
Illustrations: Ute Drewes, CH-Basel,
                          www.drewes.ch
Copyediting: Triacom Dental, D-Barendorf,
                          www.triacom-dental.de
Graphic Concept: Wirz Corporate AG, CH-Zurich
Production: Bernd Burkart, D-Berlin
Printing: Bosch-Druck GmbH, D-Landshut,
                          www.bosch-druck.de

Printed in Germany

ISBN-13: 978-3-938947-10-4
ISBN-10: 3-938947-10-1

The materials offered in the ITI Treatment Guide are for educational purposes only and intended as a step-by-step guide to treatment of a particular case and patient situation. These recommendations are based on conclusions of the ITI Consensus Conferences and, as such, in line with the ITI treatment philosophy. These recommendations, nevertheless, represent the opinions of the authors. Neither the ITI nor the authors, editors and publishers make any representation or warranty for the completeness or accuracy of the published materials and as a consequence do not accept any liability for damages (including, without limitation, direct, indirect, special, consequential or incidental damages or loss of profits) caused by the use of the information contained in the ITI Treatment Guide. The information contained in the ITI Treatment Guide cannot replace an individual assessment by a clinician, and its use for the treatment of patients is therefore in the sole responsibility of the clinician.

The inclusion of or reference to a particular product, method, technique or material relating to such products, methods, or techniques in the ITI Treatment Guide does not represent a recommendation or an endorsement of the values, features, or claims made by its respective manufacturers.

Some of the manufacturer and product names referred to in this publication may be registered trademarks or proprietary names, even though specific reference to this fact is not made. Therefore, the appearance of a name without designation as proprietary is not to be construed as a representation by the publisher that it is in the public domain.

With the exception of Fig 13a in section 4.7 and Figs 6, 7, 23, 24, 25, 27, 29, 30a, 30b, 31, 32, 33, 34, and 37 in section 5, the components of the implant system shown are part of the Straumann® Dental Implant System.

The tooth identification system used in this ITI Treatment Guide is that of the FDI World Dental Federation.

The ITI Mission is ...

"... to promote and disseminate knowledge on all aspects of implant dentistry and related tissue regeneration through research, development and education to the benefit of the patient."

Preface

In the past 15 years, the use of osseointegrated implants has become the standard of care for the rehabilitation of fully and partially edentulous patients, leading to a rapid expansion of implant therapy in dental offices.

This positive development was supported by several factors and trends. Firstly, implant therapy is meeting with much greater acceptance—not only by patients, but also by dentists. The excellent documentation of osseointegrated implants in prospective clinical studies (with up to ten years of follow-up) and good clinical results have both contributed to this increased acceptance. Secondly, the prosthodontic aspect of implant therapy has been simplified by precise prefabricated components, so general practitioners can easily treat patients with implant-supported restorations. Thirdly, there has been significant progress in bone-augmentation procedures (techniques to overcome local bone deficiencies such as guided bone regeneration or sinus grafting). These surgical procedures are routinely used for implant patients today; they have broadened the indications for oral implant therapy, particularly in partially edentulous patients.

As a result, the single-tooth replacement has become the most common indication for implant therapy in recent years. Parallel to this, "novel techniques," such as immediate implants (with or without flap elevation) and immediate loading, have been promoted to make implant therapy more patient-friendly. Most of these new techniques, however, have not yet been sufficiently documented clinically. Carefully designed, randomized, controlled clinical studies are required to evaluate their value for daily practice.

With this rapid expansion of implant therapy, involving more than 100,000 clinicians worldwide, quality control in implant dentistry has become an increasing challenge. Universities and scientific associations have been asked to make efforts to assure that the implant therapy provided is of high quality in order to maintain the good reputation of dental implants.

The International Team of Implantology (ITI) has responded by establishing the ITI Education Committee. The main objectives of this committee are to discuss and define the standards of care in the surgical and prosthetic aspects of implant dentistry, to integrate these standards into high-quality continuing-education courses, and to coordinate the worldwide educational efforts. Over the past eight years, the ITI has significantly increased its efforts in the area of implant education, including the establishment of the ITI Scholarship Program, which offers stipends to young clinicians and financial support for Centers of Implant Dentistry in the U.S., Europe, and Japan. In addition, the ITI organized its third ITI Consensus Conference in 2003 to discuss clinical topics of interest to implant dentistry. The proceedings were published in a special supplement of JOMI (Proceedings of the Third ITI Consensus Conference 2004).

The ITI Education Committee has decided to use these consensus proceedings to establish an ITI Treatment Guide. This guide will offer detailed clinical guidelines for specific problems in implant dentistry. The first volumes will discuss the following topics: (i) esthetic implant dentistry; (ii) loading protocols in implant dentistry; and (iii) implant placement in extraction sockets.

These topics will be comprehensively presented with detailed recommendations for step-by-step procedures. Each treatment option will be discussed objectively, taking into account the following parameters:

- Scientific documentation of the procedure through clinical studies
- Objective benefits for the patient
- Risks involved with the procedure
- Level of treatment complexity according to the SAC (simple—advanced—complex) classification
- Cost-effectiveness of the procedure

The first volume of the ITI Treatment Guide is devoted to single-tooth replacements in the esthetic zone, a topic of great interest within implant dentistry. It should be of great help to the clinician dealing with esthetic indications in implant patients.

Daniel Buser   Urs C. Belser   Daniel Wismeijer

Acknowledgment

The authors thank Ms. Ute Drewes for her beautiful artwork and illustrations and Dr. Kati Benthaus for her excellent support and outstanding commitment to the timely completion and high quality of this ITI Treatment Guide.

Editors and Authors

Editors:

Urs C. Belser, DMD, Professor
   University of Geneva
   Department of Prosthodontics
   School of Dental Medicine
   Rue Barthélemy-Menn 19,1211 Genève 4, Switzerland
   E-mail: urs.belser@medecine.unige.ch

Daniel Buser, DMD, Professor
   University of Berne
   Department of Oral Surgery and Stomatology
   School of Dental Medicine
   Freiburgstrasse 7, 3010 Bern, Switzerland
   E-mail: daniel.buser@zmk.unibe.ch

Daniel Wismeijer, DMD, Professor
   Academic Center for Dentistry Amsterdam (ACTA)
   Free University
   Department of Oral Function
   Section of Implantology and Prosthetic Dentistry
   Louwesweg 1, 1066 EA Amsterdam, Netherlands
   E-mail: dwismeijer@acta.nl

Authors:

Christoph Hämmerle, DMD, Professor
   University of Zurich, Center for Dental and
   Oral Medicine, Clinic for Fixed and
   Removable Prosthodontics
   Plattenstrasse 11, 8032 Zürich, Switzerland
   E-mail: hammerle@zzmk.unizh.ch

Ronald Jung, DMD
   University of Zurich, Center for Dental and
   Oral Medicine, Clinic for Fixed and
   Removable Prosthodontics
   Plattenstrasse 11, 8032 Zürich, Switzerland
   Email: jung@zzmk.unizh.ch

William C. Martin, DMD, MS
   University of Florida, Gainesville
   Center for Implant Dentistry
   Department of Oral and Maxillofacial Surgery
   1600 W Archer Road, D7-6, Gainesville, FL 32610, USA
   E-mail: wmartin@dental.ufl.edu

Dean Morton, BDS, MS
   University of Florida, Gainesville
   Center for Implant Dentistry
   Department of Oral and Maxillofacial Surgery
   1600 W Archer Road, D7-6, Gainesville, FL 32610, USA
   E-mail: dmorton@dental.ufl.edu

Bruno Schmid, DMD
   Bayweg 3, 3123 Belp, Switzerland
   E-mail: brunoschmid@vtxmail.ch

Table of Contents

1   Introduction

D. Buser, U. C. Belser, D. Wismeijer

Over the past 15 years, implant dentistry has progressed faster than many other disciplines in dental medicine. Whereas osseointegration was the primary goal two decades ago, it is nowadays taken for granted and implants are expected to remain functional for decades.

The success of implant therapy is no longer judged mainly by the osseointegration of the implant. In recent years, esthetics has become an inseparable part of oral rehabilitation as patients not only expect implant-supported restorations to be functional long-term, but also to be esthetic, especially in regions of the oral cavity that are visible when the patient smiles.

Supported by new academic curricula as well as by statements from clinical dentistry, such as the Proceedings of the Third ITI Consensus Conference published in a special 2004 supplement of JOMI, we believe that we are coming closer to creating the "perfect illusion" and maintaining it over time.

This is on one hand due to our increased knowledge of biological principles such as biologic width. On the other hand, our increasing awareness of the implementation of biomimetic principles, derived from a growing understanding of the key anatomic and optical parameters of the natural dentition, supports this goal as well.

Nevertheless, predictable optimum results in the esthetic region can only be achieved through application of a comprehensive clinical concept based on experience, sound pre-operative examination and treatment planning, and a team approach that unites patients, surgeons, prosthodontists, and dental technicians.

It is logical to use the 2004 Consensus Proceedings for drawing up and publishing detailed clinical guidelines regarding diagnosis, treatment planning, and the management of patients requiring implant therapy in the esthetic zone.

Sound, evidence-based clinical concepts that produce successful treatment outcomes are needed.

The present first volume of the ITI treatment guide provides comprehensive details on all aspects of implant therapy in the esthetic zone.

2 Proceedings of the Third ITI Consensus Conference: Esthetics in Implant Dentistry

The International Team for Implantology (ITI) is a non-profit academic organization of professionals in implant dentistry and tissue regeneration with over 2000 fellows and members in more than 40 countries. The ITI organizes consensus conferences at 5-year intervals to discuss relevant topics in implant dentistry.

The first and second ITI Consensus Conferences in 1993 and 1997 (Proceedings of the ITI Consensus Conference 2000) primarily discussed basic surgical and prosthetic issues in implant dentistry. For the Third ITI Consensus Conference in 2003, the ITI Education Committee decided to focus the discussion on four special topics that had received much attention in recent years, "Esthetics in Implant Dentistry" being one of them (Proceedings of the Third ITI Consensus Conference, published in 2004).

A working group was elected for the exploration of each topic. Working Group 2, exploring the topic of "Esthetics in Implant Dentistry," consisted of the following ITI fellows:

Group leader: Urs C. Belser

Participants: Daniel Buser
                  Jean-Paul Martinet Douteau
                  Javier G. Fabrega
                  Timothy W. Head
                  Joachim S. Hermann
                  Frank L. Higginbottom
                  John D. Jones
                  Hideaki Katsuyama
                  Scott E. Keith
                  William C. Martin
                  Stephen Rimer
                  Johannes Röckl
                  Bruno Schmid
                  Alwin Schönenberger
                  David Shafer
                  Christian ten Bruggenkate
                  Dieter Weingart

The group was asked to arrive at a consensus position related to the esthetic dimension of implant dentistry in the anterior maxilla, based on its discussion of and subsequent deliberation on three position papers that had been prepared regarding the following fields:

1. Outcome analysis of implant restorations located in the anterior maxilla
2. Anatomical and surgical considerations of implant therapy in the anterior maxilla
3. Practical prosthodontic procedures related to anterior maxillary fixed implant restorations

The subsequent text gives an overview of the consensus statements developed by the group (Belser and coworkers, 2004).

2.1 Consensus Statements and Recommended Clinical Procedures Regarding Esthetics in Implant Dentistry

In esthetic dentistry, difficulties arise in generating evidence-based statements regarding clinical procedures. Therefore, any clinical recommendations given with regard to esthetics in implant dentistry are primarily based on the expert opinion of the Esthetics consensus group. The group worked on each statement until a unanimous opinion was reached.

2.1.1 Statements A: Long-Term Results

Statement A.1
Evidence from the Literature
The use of dental implants in the esthetic zone is well documented in the literature. Numerous controlled clinical trials show that the respective overall implant survival and success rates are similar to those reported for other segments of the jaws. However, most of these studies do not include well-defined esthetic parameters.

Statement A.2
Single-Tooth Replacement
For anterior single-tooth replacement in sites without tissue deficiencies, predictable treatment outcomes, including esthetics, can be achieved because tissue support is provided by adjacent teeth.

Statement A.3
Multiple-Tooth Replacement
The replacement of multiple adjacent missing teeth in the anterior maxilla with fixed implant restorations is poorly documented. In this context, esthetic restoration is not predictable, particularly regarding the contours of the interimplant soft tissue.

Statement A.4
Newer Surgical Approaches
Currently, the literature regarding esthetic outcomes is inconclusive for the routine implementation of certain surgical approaches, such as flapless surgery and immediate or delayed implant placement with or without immediate loading in the anterior maxilla.

2.1.2 Statements B: Surgical Considerations

Statement B.1
Planning and Execution
Implant therapy in the anterior maxilla is considered an advanced or complex procedure and requires comprehensive preoperative planning and precise surgical execution based on a restoration-driven approach.

Statement B.2
Patient Selection
Appropriate patient selection is essential in achieving esthetic treatment outcomes. Treatment of high-risk patients identified through site analysis and a general risk assessment (medical status, periodontal susceptibility, smoking, and other risks) should be undertaken with caution, since esthetic results are less consistent.

Statement B.3
Implant Selection
Implant type and size should be based on site anatomy and the planned restoration. Inappropriate choice of implant body and shoulder dimensions may result in hard and/or soft tissue complications.

Statement B.4
Implant Positioning
Correct three-dimensional implant placement is essential for an esthetic treatment outcome. Respect of the comfort zones in these dimensions results in an implant shoulder located in an ideal position, allowing for an esthetic implant restoration with stable, long-term peri-implant tissue support.

Statement B.5
Soft-Tissue Stability
For long-term esthetic soft-tissue stability, sufficient horizontal and vertical bone volume is essential. When deficiencies exist, appropriate hard and/or soft-tissue augmentation procedures are required. Currently, vertical bone deficiencies are a challenge to correct and often lead to esthetic shortcomings. To optimize soft-tissue volume, complete or partial coverage of the healing cap/implant is recommended in the anterior maxilla. In certain situations, a non-submerged approach can be considered.

Medium Lip Line

Patients who exhibit a medium lip line typically display most of their anterior maxillary teeth and only very little, if any, of the supporting periodontal structures (Fig 4). Here the esthetic risk is increased and is associated with factors affecting the appearance of these teeth and restorations, such as tooth size, color, shape, texture, optical properties, relative proportions, as well as the shape and appearance of the incisal and gingival embrasures and the presence of convexity in the teeth and the surrounding structures.

High Lip Line

Patients characterized by a high lip line often display their maxillary anterior teeth in their entirety, as well as a significant portion of the supporting soft tissues (Fig 5). The esthetic risk for these patients is greatly increased, mostly associated with the gingival tissue display. It can be difficult to develop healthy, symmetric, and contoured soft tissues, and any failures will be readily visible—particularly when restoring adjacent missing teeth (Buser and coworkers, 2004). Moreover, the display of gingival structures increases the relevance of tooth proportions and their emergence profile. The esthetic contours of the gingival margins are also critical to the outcome in patients with high esthetic demands.

3.1.4 Gingival Biotype in the Treatment Area

Thick-Gingiva Biotype

A thick-gingiva biotype can be low-risk when replacing single missing teeth in the anterior area. The gingival tissues in these patients are characterized by a predominance of a thick, broad band of attached gingiva, typically resistant to recession (Cardaropoli and coworkers, 2004; Kan and coworkers, 2003; Kois and coworkers, 2001; Weisgold, 1977) (Fig 6).

The thickness of the gingival tissue effectively masks the color of the implant(s) and any subgingival metallic components, reducing the risk of not achieving a pleasing esthetic result. This biotype clearly favors the long-term stability of esthetic peri-implant soft tissues. Special surgical consideration should be given to thick-gingiva biotype patients, as they are more prone to post-surgical scarring subsequent to augmentation procedures.

For patients with multiple adjacent missing anterior teeth, a thick-tissue biotype can be both favorable and detrimental. Thick gingiva remains predictable in terms of position and appearance and resistant to recession. However, the character of the tissue reduces the likelihood of papillae developing when multi-tooth edentulous areas are present (Fig 7).

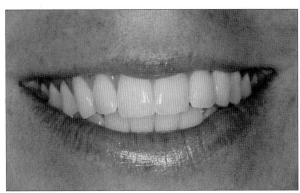

Fig 4   Medium lip line.

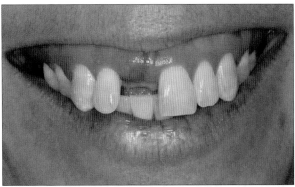

Fig 5   High lip line.

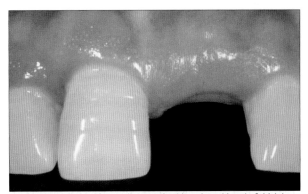

Fig 6   Thick-gingiva biotype characterized by a broad band of thick keratinized tissue and blunted papillae.

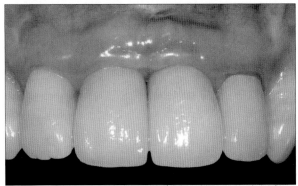

Fig 7   Restoration of adjacent spaces 11 and 21 with crowns supported by dental implants in a patient with a thick-gingiva biotype.

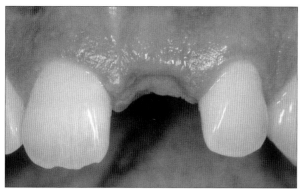

Fig 8   Medium-gingiva biotype characterized by a broad band of thin keratinized tissue with blunted papillae.

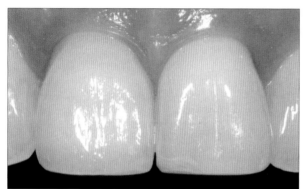

Fig 9   Restoration of a dental implant at site 11 in a patient with a thin-gingiva biotype.

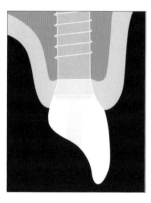

Fig 10   Slightly palatalized position of the dental implant allowing for maximum hard-tissue and soft-tissue thickness on the facial surface.

Medium-Gingiva Biotype

For patients with a medium-gingiva biotype, esthetic restoration of missing teeth is more challenging in the long term, and the esthetic risk is increased. Medium-gingiva biotypes display some characteristics of a thick biotype—most often the presence of thick attached gingival tissues. In addition, however, they can display characteristics of a thin-gingiva biotype, including long, thin, and blunted dental papillae (Fig 8).

In these cases, esthetic restorations are more challenging and less predictable over the long term.

Thin-Gingiva Biotype

A thin-gingiva biotype can be associated with excellent esthetic single-tooth restorations if the adjacent teeth are periodontally healthy and have sufficient bone-crest heights (Fig 9).

The thin and friable nature of the soft tissues is conducive to the formation and maintenance of natural and predictable interproximal dental papillae, but an increased esthetic risk is associated with the possibility of gingival recession (Cardaropoli and coworkers, 2004; Kan and coworkers, 2003; Kois and coworkers, 2001; Weisgold, 1977). Long-term predictability requires careful attention to detail with particular regard to implant position and adequate supporting bone, restoration emergence profile, and technical adaptation and contour. The health and proximity of adjacent structures as they traverse the connective tissues and epithelium is important to establishing and maintaining papillae.

The propensity for these tissues to respond to stimuli with recession cannot be ignored as a significant risk to a satisfactory esthetic outcome. Patients with adjacent missing teeth and thin-gingiva biotype often require periodontal surgery to alter the character of the tissue before or in conjunction with implant treatment. The danger of recession and tissue discoloration is further increased in patients with adjacent missing teeth, and implant position and restorative shapes become more critical.

Restorative and surgical planning for these patients requires implants to be placed closer to the palate (but still within the orofacial comfort zone), thus allowing for maximum hard-tissue and soft-tissue coverage of the dental implant surface (Buser and coworkers, 2004). This position places the long axis of the implant so that it exits through the cingulum of the restoration, favoring screw-retained restorations (Fig 10).

3.1.5 Shape of the Missing and Adjacent Teeth

The shape of the missing and adjacent teeth can profoundly influence the degree of risk associated with implant-supported restorations in the esthetic zone. With the esthetic outcome strongly influenced by the final gingival architecture, the risk can be reduced by the presence of square teeth (and, often, a thick-gingiva biotype). Although implant-supported restorations in this environment are rarely associated with long and complete papillae, it should be noted that this is often in harmony with the patient's natural state. There is little question that triangular teeth pose a greater risk and that this risk is most likely associated with the emergence anatomy and tissue support (Takei, 1980). Triangular tooth shapes often have a tissue architecture of the thin, high-scalloping type when associated with teeth in good periodontal health. A high esthetic risk is evident when a triangular tooth shape is associated with localized periodontal defects and the loss of interproximal papillae (Fig 11). These patients will often require a dental implant superstructure that is square-shaped, as well as large contact areas, potentially compromising the final appearance. When the restoration includes triangular tooth shapes, interproximal spaces (black triangles) must be anticipated.

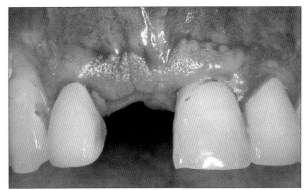

Fig 11   Pre-treatment examination. Triangular tooth shape associated with localized periodontal disease. A high esthetic risk is associated with this type of a clinical status.

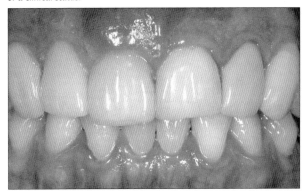

Fig 12   Acute infections at the future implant site presenting local swelling and suppuration pose maximum threat to the esthetic treatment outcome.

3.1.6 Infection at the Implant Site and Bone Level at Adjacent Teeth

The presence or history of infection, at or adjacent to an implant site, is an important consideration in the pre-operative evaluation of the esthetic risk to implant-based treatment. Local infections associated with periodontal disease, endodontic lesions, post-traumatic lesions (root fractures, root resorption, and/or ankylosis), or foreign bodies (amalgam remnants, infected root remnants), are capable of directly reducing the quantity and quality of the hard and soft tissues at potential implant sites or adjacent to them. Further, an effective treatment of the local infection, while resulting in disease resolution, can be associated with additional loss of esthetically important tissues, particularly the levels of the crestal bone on adjacent teeth or shrinkage of the soft tissues resulting in gingival recession. The characteristics of a local infection, if it is chronic or acute in nature, determines the severity of the esthetic risk subsequent to effective infection control therapy. In the context of local infections, the highest risk to an esthetic outcome is associated with acute infections demonstrating suppuration and local swelling (Fig 12). Chronic infections, in particular chronic periapical lesions of teeth to be replaced with implants, bear a medium risk for complications with esthetic significance if not resolved prior to implant placement (Lindeboom and coworkers, 2006).

For single missing teeth, the support for interproximal dental papillae is related to the height of the bone crests on adjacent teeth (Choquet and coworkers, 2001; Kan and coworkers, 2003). Therefore, the contours of the restoration (specifically the positions and extent of the contact areas), in addition to the presence of interdental papillae and the esthetic outcome, depend on the height of the crestal bone adjacent to the implant site (Fig 13). Where local infections have resulted in vertical bone loss around adjacent teeth, the risk of a compromised esthetic outcome is greatly increased (Fig 14). The probability of a space (black triangle) arising between a properly contoured restoration and the adjacent tooth increases with greater observable crestal bone loss on adjacent roots. Furthermore, the regeneration of crestal bone along a previously infected root surface is not predictable, and is unlikely with currently available treatment options.

For extended edentulous spaces with multiple missing teeth, the risk of a compromised esthetic outcome is considered high, since horizontal and/or vertical bone deficiencies are often present. The primary concern is in the interdental spaces that are not adjacent to teeth. The problem is magnified when adjacent implants are uti-

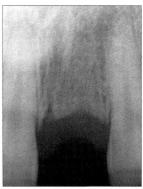 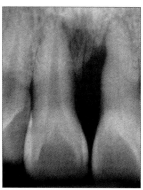

Fig 13   Radiograph showing adequate interproximal bone support.

Fig 14   Radiograph showing loss of
interproximal bone support due to
periodontal disease.

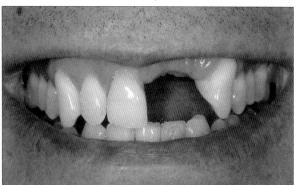

Fig 15   A high lip line, thin-gingiva biotype, and extended edentulous span
coupled with a loss of periodontal support would classify this treatment as
a maximum esthetic risk.

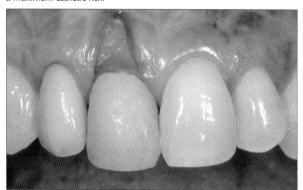

Fig 16   An existing restoration at site 12 adjacent to a future implant site
should be scheduled for replacement in conjunction with the implant
restoration.

lized in the esthetic zone, since this reduces the predictability of inter-dental closure with soft tissue (Tarnow
and coworkers, 2000; Tarnow and coworkers, 2003). When
combined with additional risk factors such as a high lip
line and/or a thin-gingiva biotype, the placement of adjacent implants in extended edentulous spaces in the anterior maxilla often represents maximum esthetic risk (Fig
15). Site development for patients in this category is often mandatory prior to or in conjunction with implant
placement. The results of such procedures vary, with horizontal augmentations often superior to those achieved
in the vertical dimension.

Identifying patients with increased risk factors for periodontal susceptibility and/or advancing or refractory periodontal disease is also critical. Literature shows increasing evidence that these patients pose potential risk to biologic complications (Ellegaard and coworkers,1997; Karroussis and coworkers, 2003). Thus, periodontal disease
must be resolved before implant therapy is initiated. Genetic swab tests have been introduced as clinical tests to
identify patients with a positive Interleukin-1 (IL-1) genotype, as these patients run a greater risk of developing periodontitis (Korman and coworkers,1997; Nieri and
coworkers, 2002; Tai and coworkers, 2002). Recent publi-
cations show a synergy for the frequency of biological
complications, when IL-1-positive patients are also heavy
smokers (Feloutzis and coworkers, 2003; Shimpuku and
coworkers, 2003; Grucia and coworkers, 2004). These patients should be identified and informed of potential esthetic complications prior to implant therapy, and should
be more rigorously followed during the maintenance period.

3.1.7   Restorative Status of Teeth Adjacent to the Edentulous Space

When teeth adjacent to an edentulous area are healthy
from a restorative perspective, no additional risk to the esthetic outcome is predicted. Adjacent teeth with restorations extending into the gingival sulcus, however, represent a serious threat. Subgingival margins are often associated with recession subsequent to the placement of an
implant, and esthetic complications can be associated
with exposed restorative margins or an altered gingival architecture (Fig 16). For these patients, meticulous treatment planning is vital and may include the replacement
of the adjacent restoration as part of the treatment, or
modification of the surgical incision to reduce risk.

3.1.8 Character of the Edentulous Space

The chances of an esthetic treatment outcome are higher for single missing teeth (Belser and coworkers, 1996; Belser and coworkers, 2000; Belser and coworkers, 2004). The neighboring teeth and supporting structures, however, must be in good health. There is a clearly lower esthetic risk if support for the gingival tissue is provided by the proximal crests of bone on adjacent teeth and if the distance from this bone to the restoration's contact points above is short (Kan and coworkers, 2003). The esthetic result can be compromised when the edentulous site is associated with unfavorable periodontal conditions or inadequate restorative space.

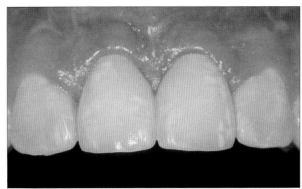

Fig 17   When redundant tissue is present in the nasopalatine area, restoration of adjacent dental implants may lead to an acceptable result.

Consensus Statement A.2
Single-Tooth Replacement:
For anterior single-tooth replacements in sites without tissue deficiencies, predictable treatment outcomes, including esthetics, can be achieved because tissue support is provided by adjacent teeth.

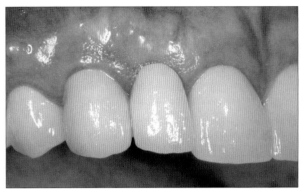

Fig 18   A mesially cantilevered restoration from a dental implant at sites 13 and 12.

Clinically, adjacent missing teeth greatly increases the esthetic challenge. Inter-implant soft-tissue and hard-tissue support becomes unpredictable because the morphology of the implants may cause the coronal aspect of the osseous crest between them to decrease (Buser and coworkers, 2004; Tarnow and coworkers, 2003). For this reason, the restoration-based placement of dental implants to allow for maximum inter-implant tissue support is paramount; even small errors can be detrimental. The planning of implant treatment for these patients should consider the increased risk posed by adjacent implants and the need for surgical precision. Appropriate implant selection is imperative, as the use of oversized implants can result in increased bone attrition and consequent facial and proximal tissue loss (Buser and coworkers, 2004).

The location of the adjacent missing teeth is important to the assessment of the esthetic risk. Missing central incisors provide the best opportunity for an esthetic result due to potential "redundant" tissue located in the nasopalatine area, and the symmetry of gingival architecture required after healing (Fig 17).

When replacing adjacent central and lateral incisors, the challenge is increased by the need to provide anatomically correct gingival zenith positions. Further, the emergence of appropriately contoured adjacent restorations through the connective tissue is critical if papillary support is to be gained, increasing the reliance on appropriate implant selection (size and shape). The restoration of

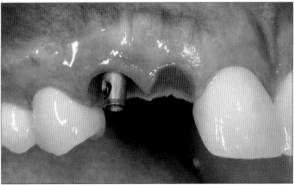

Fig 19   An ovate pontic created at site 12 to help maximize interproximal tissue support.

lateral incisors and canines presents the same difficulties. Treatment options should be explored to prevent the placement of adjacent implants in these areas where possible. In general, when a lateral incisor is involved adjacent to a missing central incisor or canine, a cantilevered restoration into the lateral site should be considered (Fig 18).

This will allow the implant team to capitalize on a single implant position while creating an ovate pontic into the lateral site, potentially maximizing interproximal tissue support (Fig 19).

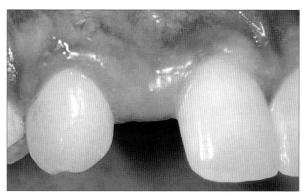

Fig 20a   Frontal view of a missing lateral incisor highlighting excess vertical height of soft tissue.

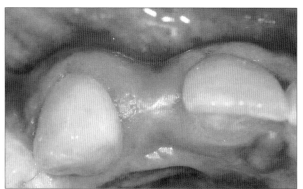

Fig 20b   Occlusal view of the missing lateral incisor highlighting deficient horizontal width of hard tissue.

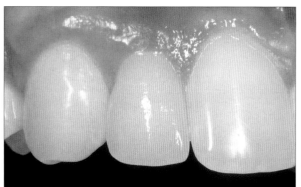

Fig 20c   Replacement of the missing lateral incisor with a dental implant and ceramo-metal restoration.

Patients who exhibit adjacent missing teeth including a lateral incisor should be considered as having a maximum risk of esthetic complications when adjacent implants are utilized.

3.1.9   Width of the Hard and Soft Tissues in the Edentulous Space

Tissue deficiencies in the horizontal dimension can pose an increased esthetic treatment risk. The risk can be low if adjacent structures are healthy and if extractions (where required) are performed with a minimum of trauma to the bone and surrounding soft tissues. If the defect is restricted to the horizontal dimension and other conditions are satisfied (such as the periodontal and restorative integrity of the adjacent teeth), site enhancement is predictable, and an esthetic outcome can be expected (Hämmerle and coworkers, 2003; Hermann and Buser, 1996) (Figs 20a-c).

The risk of a compromised esthetic outcome increases with the degree of horizontal bone loss and non-enhanced sites. In such cases, bone and soft-tissue height is compromised by deeper implant placement, which is undertaken to provide increased ridge width. Deeper implant placement can also be detrimental to esthetics as the proportions of the restorations, and their emergence profiles, are negatively influenced (Buser and coworkers, 2004). Such situations can often be effectively addressed with site enhancement through horizontal bone augmentation and/or soft-tissue grafting (Jemt and coworkers, 1997; Salama and coworkers, 1996). These procedures have been improved greatly in recent years and offer a high degree of predictability in sites with horizontal deficiencies.

Consensus Statement B.5
Soft-Tissue Stability:
For long-term esthetic soft-tissue stability, sufficient horizontal and vertical bone volume is essential. When deficiencies exist, appropriate hard and/or soft tissue augmentation procedures are required. Currently, vertical bone deficiencies are a challenge to correct and often lead to esthetic shortcomings. To optimize soft tissue volume, complete or partial coverage of the healing cap/implant is recommended in the anterior maxilla. In certain situations, a non-submerged approach can be considered.

3.1.10 Height of the Hard and Soft Tissues in the Edentulous Space

Small deficiencies in vertical bone height greatly increase the risk of not achieving an esthetic outcome, as augmentation procedures are still not entirely predictable (Fig 21a). Under most circumstances, regenerative procedures increase the width of the implant sites but do not recapture adequate height. This results in a compromised gingival and restorative appearance (Fig 21b).

Loss of vertical bone in the edentulous space also magnifies the risk associated with many other factors—particularly the periodontal health of adjacent teeth. Vertically deficient sites that border on periodontally involved teeth cannot be enhanced without addressing the periodontal disease itself. Grafting adjuncts (enamel matrix proteins) should be considered as a means of restoring periodontal support in conjunction with the onlay graft (Francetti and coworkers, 2005). When periodontally compromised teeth are involved in future implant sites, tooth extrusion should be considered (Salama and coworkers, 1996).

Patients who exhibit vertical hard-tissue or soft-tissue loss are associated with a high esthetic risk. When vertical deficiencies are present in adjacent edentulous areas, localized grafting techniques (distraction, onlay, free gingival grafts) should be seriously considered; the maximum esthetic risk applies.

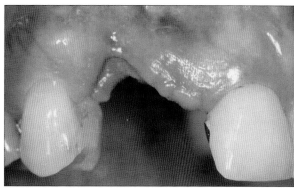

Fig 21a   Frontal view of a missing canine and lateral incisor highlighting a vertical bone deficiency.

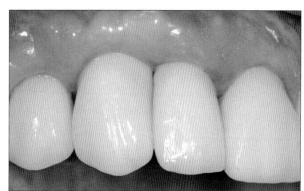

Fig 21b   Frontal view of the final restorations on dental implants.

Consensus Statement B.5
Soft-Tissue Stability:
For long-term esthetic soft-tissue stability, sufficient horizontal and vertical bone volume is essential. When deficiencies exist, appropriate hard and/or soft tissue augmentation procedures are required. Currently, vertical bone deficiencies are a challenge to correct and often lead to esthetic shortcomings. To optimize soft tissue volume, complete or partial coverage of the healing cap/implant is recommended in the anterior maxilla. In certain situations, a non-submerged approach can be considered.

3.1.11 Esthetic Risk Profile: Summary

Table 2 summarizes the various risk factors. The individual risk profile of each patient is established based on a detailed preoperative analysis. The use of this esthetic risk profile table will be exemplified in sections 4.4 through 4.14 for specific patient cases.

Table 2 Esthetic risk assessment for edentulous sites.

Esthetic Risk Factors	Low	Medium	High
Medical status	Healthy patient and intact immune system		Reduced immune system
Smoking habit	Non-smoker	Light smoker (< 10 cig/d)	Heavy smoker (> 10 cig/d)
Patient's esthetic expectation	Low	Medium	High
Lip line	Low	Medium	High
Gingival biotype	Low-scalloped, thick	Medium-scalloped, medium-thick	High-scalloped, thin
Shape of tooth crowns	Rectangular		Triangular
Infection at implant site	None	Chronic	Acute
Bone level at adjacent teeth	≤ 5 mm to contact point	5.5 to 6.5 mm to contact point	≥ 7 mm to contact point
Restorative status of neighboring teeth	Virgin		Restored
Width of edentulous span	1 tooth (≥ 7 mm)[1] 1 tooth (≥ 5.5 mm)[2]	1 tooth (< 7 mm)[1] 1 tooth (< 5.5 mm)[2]	2 teeth or more
Soft-tissue anatomy	Intact soft tissue		Soft-tissue defects
Bone anatomy of alveolar crest	Alveolar crest without bone deficiency	Horizontal bone deficiency	Vertical bone deficiency

[1] *Standard Plus implants, Regular Neck*   [2] *Standard Plus implants, Narrow Neck*

3.2 Treatment Planning

The esthetic risk profile will help minimize potential restorative pitfalls that may ultimately be associated with unacceptable restorative outcomes. While the restoration itself can be enhanced by the expertise of the dental technician through office-laboratory communication, it is necessary for the restorative dentist to have a clear understanding of the materials and techniques involved in enhancing the soft-tissue response around the restoration. The anatomy of the transition zone (the emergence profile created from the shoulder of the implant to the mucosal margin) will play a large role in the contours of the definitive restoration and the effects it has on peri-implant tissue support (Figs 22a, b).

In most situations, the anatomy of the transition zone around anterior implants poses a challenge when creating access to the shoulder of the ideally placed implant. It is not uncommon to find an implant 2 mm submucosal at the mid-facial aspect and 5 – 6 mm submucosal at the interproximal aspect. Limited access to the shoulder in the interproximal region makes it difficult to justify placement of a cement line at the implant shoulder. Cement trapped in the submucosa can lead to peri-implant inflammation and in extreme cases to the loss of bone substance on the implant surface. In these clinical situations, placing a machined margin at shoulder level to help reduce potential inflammation is recommended (Belser and coworkers, 2004). Restorative options in these situations include a screw-retained restoration or a customized abutment (metal, ceramo-metal, ceramic) to allow for the cement line to be placed closer to the mucosal margin for better access (Higginbottom and coworkers, 2004). In occasional clinical situations, the implant shoulders may be located 2 – 3 mm submucosal around the entire circumference of the implant (Fig 23). These patients can benefit from a cemented or screw-retained restoration.

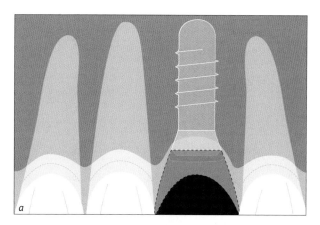

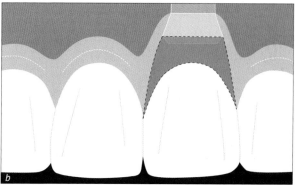

Figs 22a, b   The transition zone (red) is the area located between the shoulder of the implant and the mucosal margin.

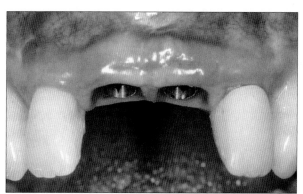

Fig 23   A circumferential implant shoulder depth of less than 2 – 3 mm would allow for access to a cement line on the shoulder of the implants.

3.3 Interim Restorations

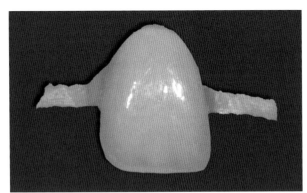

Fig 24a   Laboratory-processed fiber-reinforced fixed partial denture.

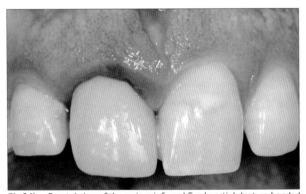

Fig 24b   Frontal view of the resin-reinforced fixed partial denture bonded in place immediately following extraction of tooth 11.

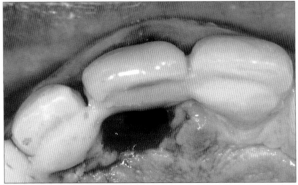

Fig 24c   Occlusal view of the resin-reinforced fixed partial denture in place highlighting the flowable composite used to anchor it in place.

The treatment of edentulous spans in the esthetic zone that have pre-existing soft-tissue and/or hard-tissue deficiencies will require surgical augmentation procedures before or in conjunction with implant placement. These procedures will often require a healing phase before the seating of provisional restorations on dental implants. A well-designed interim restoration will not only provide esthetic relief for the patient, but will help protect the tissue as it matures during the healing phase (Markus, 1999).

Interim restorations can be either fixed or removable. Both options can provide benefits for the patient, but certain key principles should be followed to prevent deleterious effects on the tissue in the edentulous space (Buser and coworkers, 2004). Interim restorations must:

1. Satisfy (within reason) the patient's esthetic expectations.
2. Be easy to fabricate and maintain.
3. Eliminate intermittent vertical pressure.
4. Be durable.
5. Provide diagnostic value.

When vertical site enhancement procedures are performed, it is necessary to design an interim restoration that eliminates vertical intermittent pressure. Removable prostheses that rely on the palatal tissue for retention and resistance can create undesirable pressure in the area, causing vertical loss of the graft. Designing an interim restoration that will eliminate these pressures is recommended.

Options for ideal interim restorations:

1. *Fixed partial denture* – If teeth adjacent to the edentulous site are scheduled for full coverage restorations, this interim prosthesis can provide good esthetics and function while the site matures.
2. *Resin fiber-reinforced fixed partial denture* – If interocclusal space permits, a denture tooth with fiber wings can be bonded to the palatal surface of adjacent teeth, providing an esthetic fixed alternative (Figs 24a-c). Alternative procedures utilizing small interproximal retention preparations (within enamel) can be performed to retain a denture tooth with composite resin.
3. *Orthodontics* – Patients undergoing orthodontic treatment or patients who accept the utilization of brackets to retain a rectangular wire and a pontic can benefit from a low-maintenance, easily retrievable fixed alternative.
4. *Vacuform retainer* – If interocclusal space is limited and orthodontic treatment is not an option, a vacuform retainer with an ovate pontic can provide an interim restoration that will have controllable pressure on the graft site (Moskowitz and coworkers, 1997) (Fig 25). Vacuform retainers are not recommended for extended use, since occlusal interference and excessive denture wear must be expected.
5. *Removable partial denture (RPD)* – Patients can benefit from a removable prosthesis when a vertical deficiency does not exist. An acrylic-resin RPD gains its support from the palatal tissue and allows for the pontic to be designed in an ovate form for tissue shaping (Figs 26a, b).

When needed, extra retention can be added by using interproximal wrought-wire ball clasps. RPDs are not recommended if vertical grafting is planned. The potential exists for intermittent pressure on the grafted site (even when relieved), which could lead to resorption.

An interim restoration that meets these recommendations is an esthetic and functional prosthesis that at the same time protects the site undergoing enhancement procedures.

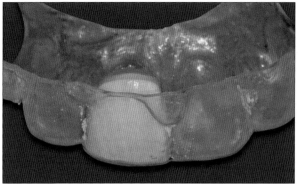

Fig 25   Vacuform retainer with a retained extracted tooth modified to an ovate form.

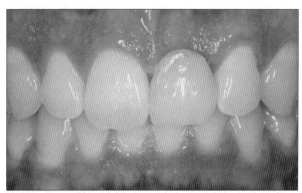

Fig 26a   Removable partial denture replacing tooth 21 in a patient who require's horizontal augmentation in conjunction with implant placement.

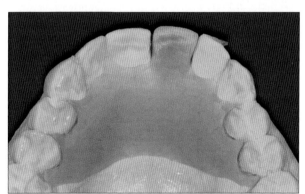

Fig 26b   Occlusal view of a resin-based removable partial denture utilizing the embrasures between the posterior teeth for retention.

3.4 Conclusions

Careful and consistent site analysis can often alert clinicians and patients to the degree of esthetic risk associated with dental treatment, allowing the dentist and, above all, the patient to develop reasonable treatment expectations. The assessment of the esthetic risk, in conjunction with an assessment of the importance the patient assigns to the esthetic outcome, are essential for improving the quality and predictability of treatment results.

4 <u>Achieving Optimal Esthetic Results</u>

4.1 Surgical Considerations for Single-Tooth Replacements in the Esthetic Zone: Standard Procedure in Sites Without Bone Deficiencies

D. Buser, W. C. Martin, U. C. Belser

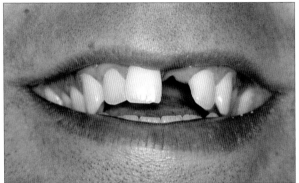

Fig 1   The patient's smile, revealing a high lip line situation.

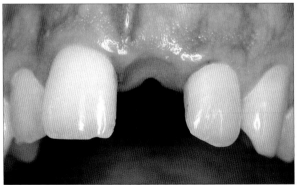

Fig 2   Single-tooth gap caused by a dental trauma. Edentulous span and alveolar crest adequately dimensioned for implant therapy.

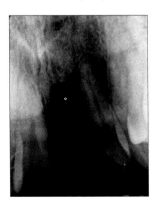

Fig 3   Periapical radiograph showing normal bone structures in the edentulous gap.

The following case demonstrates the general principles of implant placement in the esthetic zone:

The patient had a missing upper left central incisor, which he had lost by trauma. At full natural smile, the patient exhibited a high lip line situation and a harmoniously scalloped gingival margin (Fig 1).

The tissue biotype was thin and highly scalloped (Fig 2). In general, the combination of a high lip line and a thin-gingiva biotype is considered a high-risk situation from an anatomic point of view. Patients with such a risk profile should be treated with caution.

The periapical radiograph of the single-tooth gap, taken in May 1996, demonstrated adequate bone height and the absence of pathological processes (Fig 3).

Consensus Statement B.2
Patient Selection:
Appropriate patient selection is essential in achieving esthetic treatment outcomes. Treatment of high-risk patients identified through site analysis and a general risk assessment (medical status, periodontal susceptibility, smoking, and other risks) should be undertaken with caution, since esthetic results are less consistent.

Consensus Statement B.1
Planning and Execution:
Implant therapy in the anterior maxilla is considered an advanced or complex procedure and requires comprehensive preoperative planning and precise surgical execution based on a restoration-driven approach.

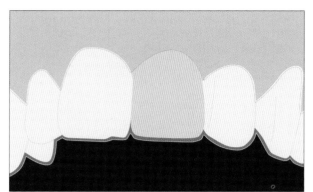

Fig 4 Schematic diagram of a waxup that can be used for the fabrication of a surgical template.

In complex cases, a diagnostic waxup can be beneficial as a basis for fabricating a surgical template (Fig 4), which facilitates correct three-dimensional implant placement during surgery. Here, the cervical end of the template in the tooth-gap position indicated the desired future soft-tissue margin at the implant-supported crown.

Esthetic implant placement is based upon a restoration-driven philosophy. Correct three-dimensional implant positioning will allow for optimal support and the stability of the peri-implant hard and soft tissues (Buser and coworkers, 2004).

Consensus Statement B.3
Implant Selection:
Implant type and size should be based on site anatomy and the planned restoration. Inappropriate choice of implant body and shoulder dimensions may result in hard and/or soft tissue complications.

In the anterior maxilla, the implant types of the Straumann Dental Implant System shown in Table 1 are recommended for clinical use.

These implants differ in restorative shoulder diameter and endosseous diameter. To use these implants successfully in the anterior maxilla, correct implant selection relative to the mesiodistal dimension of the tooth to be replaced (gap size) is critical (Table 2).

Table 1 Implant types recommended for use in the anterior maxilla (Straumann Dental Implant System)

Implant	Description
	Standard Plus implant Endosseous ⌀ 4.1 mm Regular Neck (⌀ 4.8 mm)
	Standard Plus implant Endosseous ⌀ 4.8 mm Regular Neck (⌀ 4.8 mm)
	Standard Plus implant Endosseous ⌀ 3.3 mm Narrow Neck (⌀ 3.5 mm)
	Tapered Effect implant Endosseous ⌀ 4.1 mm Regular Neck (⌀ 4.8 mm)
	Tapered Effect implant Endosseous ⌀ 3.3 mm Regular Neck (⌀ 4.8 mm)

Table 2 Relationship between the mesiodistal gap size and the diameter of the implant shoulder (Straumann Dental Implant System)

Implant Type	Shoulder Diameter (mm)	Minimum Gap Size (mm)	Ideal Gap Size (mm)
Implants with a Regular Neck (⌀ 4.8 mm)	4.8	7.0	8.0–9.0
Implants with a Narrow Neck (⌀ 3.5 mm)	3.5	5.5	6.0–7.0

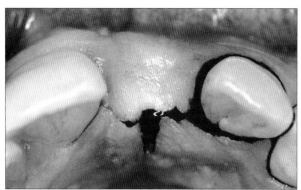

Fig 5   Occlusal view of the crestal incision, which is positioned 2 – 3 mm palatally.

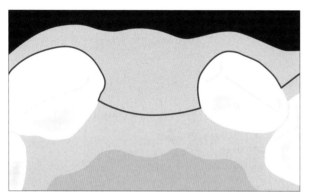

Fig 6   Schematic drawing of the crestal incision.

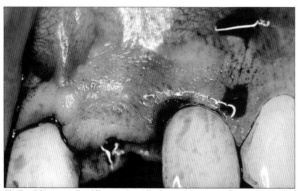

Fig 7   Divergent distal line angles relieving incisions are often used to allow the incision of the periosteum and subsequent tension-free primary soft-tissue closure.

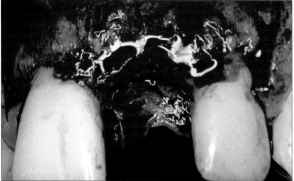

Fig 8   Clinical status following flap elevation.

Wide Neck implants, with their 6.5-mm shoulder diameter, are not recommended for use in the anterior maxilla. Their implant shoulder margin is likely to be located too close to adjacent teeth or too far facially, encroaching on their respective danger zones.

Under local anesthesia, a full thickness flap was created with a crestal incision located approximately 2 – 3 mm toward the palatal aspect (Figs 5, 6). The relieving incisions were placed at the distal line angles of the neighboring teeth.

The flap was extended through the sulcus of the adjacent teeth, ascending to the facial aspect of the alveolar crest with divergent distal line angle relieving incisions (Figs 7, 8). These incisions avoid the formation of scar tissue in the mid-crestal area and ensure sufficient vascularization of the facial flap, especially in the area of the future papillae.

Alternatively, a para-papillary incision technique could have been used.

The facial and palatal mucoperiosteal flaps were elevated with a fine tissue elevator to allow low-trauma soft-tissue handling.

Following flap elevation, the surgical site was carefully analyzed. Special attention was paid to the evaluation of the facial aspect of the alveolar crest, since sufficient bone volume in this area is an important prerequisite for an esthetic treatment outcome (Fig 8).

A periodontal probe was placed on the facial surface of adjacent teeth to examine if the facial bone wall was flattened in relation to adjacent teeth (Fig 9). Furthermore, in implant sites in the central incisor area, the location of the nasopalatal foramen needed to be determined.

A bone-scalloping procedure was performed in order to facilitate an easier and more precise preparation of the implant bed (Fig 10).

The scalloping procedure smoothens the alveolar crest and imitates its natural shape. This helps visualize and control the optimal implant position and facilitates precise implant-bed preparation.

Consensus Statement A.2
Single-Tooth Replacement:
For anterior single-tooth replacement in sites without tissue deficiencies, predictable treatment outcomes, including esthetics, can be achieved because tissue support is provided by adjacent teeth.

No bone should be removed in the proximal area of the adjacent teeth, because this bone is important for the support and maintenance of the papillae (Fig 11).

Although not mandatory for implant placement in single-tooth gaps, the use of surgical templates in the anterior maxilla can be valuable for properly placing the implant shoulder in a position that will allow for an ideal emergence profile and long-term peri-implant hard-tissue and soft-tissue support (Higginbottom and Wilson, 1996). A diagnostic waxup highlighting the final gingival margin position, facial surface, and embrasure form of the proposed restoration indicates these positions and should be the basis for generation of the surgical template. The template imitates the future soft-tissue margin at the implant crown (Fig 12).

Furthermore, the spiral drill is guided by the surgical template for proper alignment of the implant.

After implant placement, the implant shoulder was located in the desired, formerly planned position about 2 mm apical to the future soft-tissue margin around the implant-supported crown (Fig 12).

The placement of implants in a correct three-dimensional position is one of the keys to an esthetic treatment outcome, regardless of the implant system used. The correct three-dimensional position is dependent upon the planned restoration that the implant will support (Belser and coworkers, 1996; Belser and coworkers, 1998; Buser and von Arx, 2000). The relationship of the position between the implant and the proposed restoration should be based upon the position of the implant shoulder, since it will influence the final hard and soft tissue response. The implant shoulder position can be viewed in three dimensions:

1. Mesiodistal
2. Orofacial
3 Coronoapical

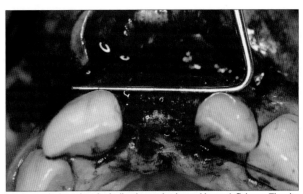

Fig 9   Periodontal probe indicating no horizontal bone deficiency. The site did not require horizontal bone augmentation.

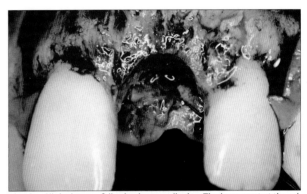

Fig 10   Clinical status following bone scalloping. The bone crest at the adjacent teeth is not touched.

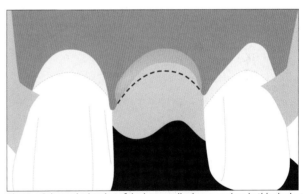

Fig 11   Schematic drawing of the bone scalloping procedure in this single-tooth gap.

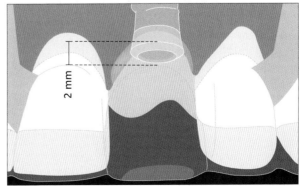

Fig 12   The future soft tissue margin at the implant crown as imitated by the template served to place the implant shoulder in the ideal position.

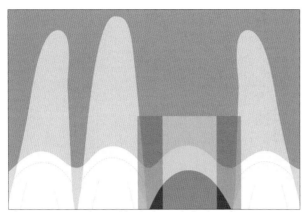

Fig 13   Correct implant position in the mesiodistal comfort zone (green).

When planning for an ideal three-dimensional implant position, a distinction is made between "comfort" and "danger" zones in each dimension (Buser and coworkers, 2004). The selection of the implant type and the placement of the dental implant should be based on the restorations planned in these zones. If implant shoulders are positioned within the danger zones, complications such as peri-implant bone resorption followed by soft-tissue recession may occur, resulting in esthetic complications. Implants positioned in the comfort zones provide the basis for a long-term stable esthetic restoration. Comfort and danger zones are defined in the mesiodistal, orofacial, and coronoapical dimensions.

4.1.1   Mesiodistal Dimension

In the mesiodistal dimension, the danger zones (red color) are located next to the adjacent root surfaces. This danger zone is about 1.0 – 1.5 mm wide (Fig 13).

With the tulip shape of the implant shoulder on Straumann implants, this places the implant body surface no closer than 1.5 mm to the adjacent root surfaces.

Proper mesiodistal implant placement avoids the danger zones adjacent to the neighboring teeth (Figs 14, 15).

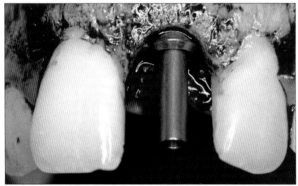

Fig 14   Status following implant insertion. The implant shoulder is positioned in the comfort zone.

Placing the implant shoulder too close to an adjacent tooth can cause the resorption of the interproximal alveolar crest to the level of that of the implant (Esposito and coworkers, 1993). With the loss of the interproximal crest height comes a reduction in papillary height. This also creates restorative problems: poor embrasure forms and emergence profiles will result in restorations with long contact zones and a compromised clinical outcome. The loss of crest height at adjacent teeth is caused by the bone saucerization routinely found around the implant shoulder of osseointegrated implants. Bone loss occurs in both the horizontal and vertical dimensions, creating a circumferential bone saucer around the implant.

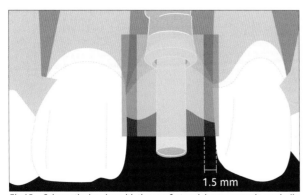

1.5 mm

Fig 15   Schematic drawing with the comfort and danger zones in mesiodistal direction.

Because the horizontal dimension of this resorption area measures about 1.0 – 1.5 mm from the implant surface (Fig 16), this minimal distance needs to be respected at implant placement to prevent vertical bone loss on adjacent teeth.

With regard to the coronoapical position of the implant shoulder, the vertical dimension of the bone saucer will lead to undesired bone loss if the implant is placed too far apically. When measured from the microgap, this vertical dimension amounts to approximately 2 mm (Hermann and coworkers, 1997; Hermann and coworkers, 2000) in interproximal areas (Fig 17). This may affect the height of the facial bone wall as well and can lead to undesired soft-tissue recession in this extremely important esthetic zone.

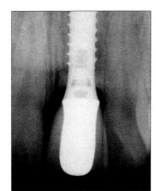 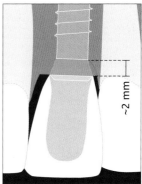

Fig 16   The typical radiographic appearance of a bone saucer around a Straumann implant with a vertical and a horizontal component.

Fig 17   Schematic drawing of the radiographic appearance of a bone saucer around a Straumann implant.

4.1.2   Orofacial Dimension

In the orofacial dimension, the implant shoulder should be positioned in the comfort zone (green color). The comfort zone measures about 1.5 – 2.0 mm in width when measured from the ideal point of emergence. The danger zones (red color) are located both facially and palatally to the comfort zone (Fig 18).

The facial danger zone is entered when the implant is placed too far facially, i.e. facially of an imaginary line connecting the point of emergence of adjacent teeth. An implant in the facial danger zone will result in the potential risk of soft-tissue recession, since the thickness of the facial bone wall is clearly reduced by the malpositioned implant. In addition, potential prosthetic complications could result in restoration – implant axis problems, making the implant difficult to restore.

The palatal danger zone is entered when the implant is placed more than 2 mm palatal to this imaginary line, since this implant position often results in a restoration with a ridge-lap design (Belser and coworkers, 1998).

After the implant bed is prepared, the facial bone wall should be intact. It should ideally measure at least 2 mm in thickness. This is important to ensure proper soft-tissue support and to avoid the resorption of the facial bone wall following restoration (Fig 19).

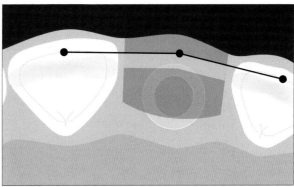

Fig 18   Schematic drawing of the orofacial comfort and danger zones.

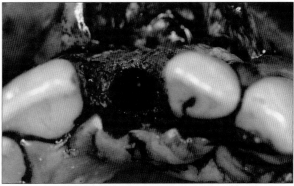

Fig 19   Occlusal view following implant bed preparation with a proper orofacial implant position and an intact facial bone wall.

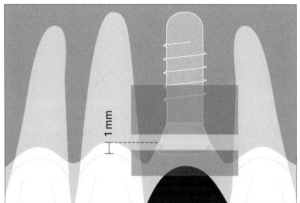

Fig 20   Periodontal probe visualizing the correct position of the implant shoulder in orofacial direction.

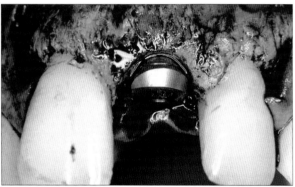

Fig 21   Comfort and danger zones in the coronoapical dimension.

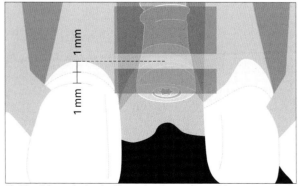

Fig 22   Correct implant placement in a coronoapical direction.

Fig 23   Schematic drawing illustrating the comfort and danger zones in the coronoapical dimension.

The implant shoulder should be positioned in the orofacial comfort zone. (Fig 20).

4.1.3   Coronoapical Dimension

In the coronoapical dimension, the comfort zone is a narrow band of about 1 mm. Ideally, the shoulder of a Straumann implant should be positioned about 1 mm apical to the cemento-enamel junction (CEJ) of the contralateral tooth (Buser and von Arx, 2000; Buser and coworkers, 2004). This recommendation, however, is only valid for teeth without periodontal tissue loss (Fig 21).

This ideally results in an implant shoulder located approximately 2 mm apical to the mid-facial gingival margin of the implant restoration (Figs 22, 23).

This can be accomplished through a surgical template highlighting the gingival margin of the planned restoration (Higginbottom and Wilson, 1996).

In patients without vertical tissue deficiencies, the use of a periodontal probe leveled on the adjacent CEJs in single-tooth gaps has proven to be a valid alternative (Buser and von Arx, 2000).

It is important to note that the CEJ of adjacent teeth can vary depending on the tooth to be replaced, and must be taken into consideration. In particular, lateral incisors are smaller and their CEJ is normally located more coronally compared to the CEJ of central incisors or canines. Implant placement within the apical danger zone (located anywhere 3 mm or further apically of the proposed gingival margin) can result in undesired facial bone resorption and subsequent gingival recession. The coronal danger zone is invaded with a supragingival shoulder position leading to a visible metal margin and poor emergence profile.

The use of a short, beveled healing cap facilitated a tension-free adaptation of the facial flap over the implant site towards the palatal aspect (Fig 24).

In patients without local bone defects and no need for bone grafting procedures, soft-tissue grafting can be used to improve the thickness and contour of the facial mucosa.

Consensus Statement B.5
Soft-Tissue Stability:
For long-term esthetic soft-tissue stability, sufficient horizontal and vertical bone volume is essential. When deficiencies exist, appropriate hard and/or soft tissue augmentation procedures are required. Currently, vertical bone deficiencies are a challenge to correct and often lead to esthetic shortcomings. To optimize soft tissue volume, complete or partial coverage of the healing cap/implant is recommended in the anterior maxilla. In certain situations, a non-submerged approach can be considered.

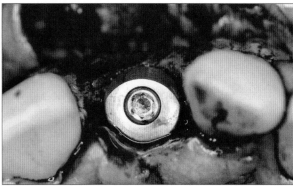

Fig 24   Occlusal view of the implant site with the inserted implant and a beveled healing cap.

If required, a free connective-tissue graft can be used from the palate at implant placement (Figs 25, 26). As implants are increasingly placed into non-healed extraction sockets, the frequency of soft tissue grafting has dropped significantly in the past five years, whereas more and more implants in the esthetic zone are placed in combination with a simultaneous guided bone regeneration (GBR) procedure.

Returning to our case, the graft was placed on the facial aspect of the implant site in order to check its shape and position (Fig 27).

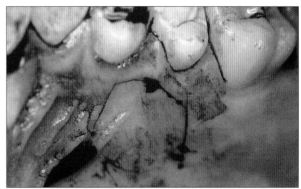

Fig 25   Harvesting site opened with a mucosal incision in the premolar area of the palate.

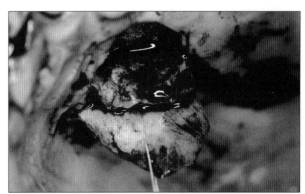

Fig 26   Harvesting a small connective-tissue graft following elevation of a mucosal flap.

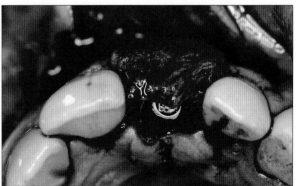

Fig 27   Positioning the connective-tissue graft.

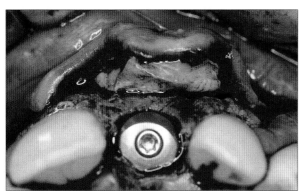

Fig 28   Occlusal view demonstrating the soft-tissue graft sutured to the mucoperiosteal flap.

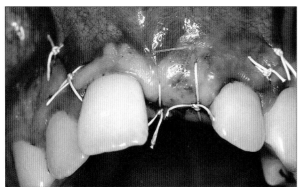

Fig 29   Status following a tension-free primary wound closure.

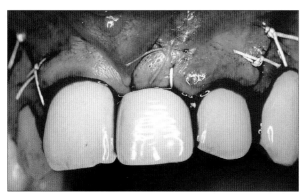

Fig 30   Insertion of the shortened partial denture after completion of surgery.

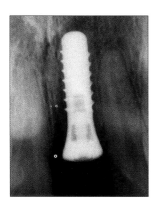

Fig 31   Post-surgical radiograph indicating a correct implant position.

The graft was sutured to the periosteum of the mucoperiosteal flap to avoid displacement during wound closure (Fig 28). Suturing also ensured close and secure contact with the facial flap, thus facilitating proper vascularization.

In most cases, the incision of the periosteum is necessary to mobilize the flap coronally, and to obtain a tension-free primary wound closure using 5-0 and 6-0 non-resorbable, atraumatic suture material (Fig 29).

The mucoperiosteal flap was precisely repositioned for submerged healing. Precise repositioning of the flap margins is especially important in the area of the future papillae.

After surgery, the existing partial denture was shortened and put in place (Fig 30).

The provisional restoration should not exert any pressure on the soft tissues. In general, interim restorations that are fixed to adjacent teeth are more beneficial for implant integration and soft-tissue maintenance, since they eliminate the possibility for undesired soft-tissue contact. They, however, are more difficult to handle for the clinician.

Following surgery, a periapical radiograph was taken to examine the position and direction of the implant and its relationship to the roots of adjacent teeth (Fig 31).

During the soft-tissue healing period of two to three weeks, chemical plaque control with chlorhexidine digluconate (0.1%) is normally performed. Follow-up visits are recommended after 7, 14, and 21 days.

After six weeks, bone healing for implants with an SLA (Sandblasted, Large-grit, Acid-etched) surface will have sufficiently progressed in standard sites without peri-implant bone defects. In implant sites where a simultaneous bone-augmentation procedure was performed, a healing period of eight to twelve weeks is required, depending on the extent and morphology of the bone defect present at the time of implant placement.

The restorative phase started after soft-tissue healing and successful osseointegration of the implant.

Consensus Statement A.4
Newer Surgical Approaches:
Currently, the literature regarding esthetic outcomes is inconclusive for the routine implementation of certain surgical approaches, such as flapless surgery and immediate or delayed implant placement with or without immediate loading in the anterior maxilla.

At the completion of bone healing, the soft tissues were healthy. The soft tissue in the implant site displayed an excellent convex contour and favorable color (Fig 32).

The implant site was reopened with a punch technique using a 12b blade to gain access to the implant shoulder. Following removal of the short healing cap, a long healing cap was inserted to establish a soft-tissue "tunnel" from the implant shoulder to the soft-tissue surface (Fig 33).

Instead of a long healing cap, a provisional restoration may be instantly inserted using a chairside technique to initiate the important phase of soft-tissue conditioning.

A few days after reopening, the soft tissues had healed uneventfully so that the restorative phase could be started (Fig 34).

For impression-taking, the use of a screw-retained transfer system is recommended in esthetic sites to ensure a precise and reproducible transfer of the implant position from the mouth to the master cast.

An acrylic-resin provisional crown, based on a prefabricated screw-retained titanium post for temporary restorations, ensured the shaping of esthetic peri-implant soft-tissue contours.

The periapical radiograph demonstrates the precise seating of the screw-retained provisional crown (Fig 35).

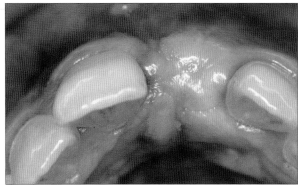

Fig 32   Occlusal view of the implant site before the reopening procedure.

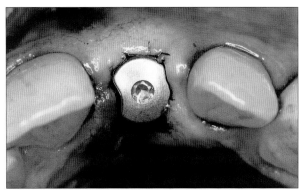

Fig 33   Status following the reopening procedure and insertion of a long titanium healing cap.

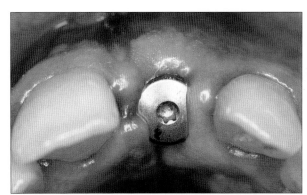

Fig 34   Clinical status a few days after the reopening procedure.

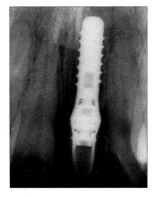

Fig 35   The periapical radiograph shows a good fit between the implant and the screw-retained provisional restoration.

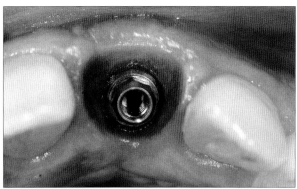

Fig 36   Occlusal view with nicely shaped peri-implant soft tissue.

The phase of soft-tissue conditioning usually takes three to six months. Before the insertion of the final implant-supported superstructure, the peri-implant soft tissue should present optimal three-dimensional contours.

In this patient, the provisional crown remained in place for three months to create ideal contours (Figs 36, 37). The final treatment outcome with a screw-retained ceramo-metal crown was pleasing for the patient, and integrated harmoniously into the natural dentition (Fig 38). The periapical radiograph demonstrated stable peri-implant bone crest levels (Fig 39).

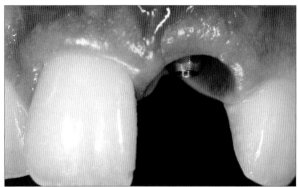

Fig 37   Facial view with nicely scalloped gingival margin.

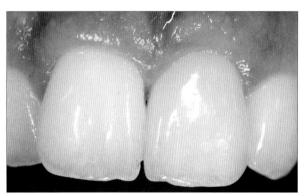

Fig 38   Esthetically pleasing treatment outcome with the implant-supported ceramo-metal crown.

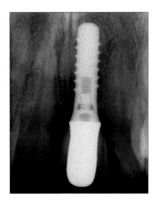

Fig 39   Periapical radiograph showing excellent precision between the implant and the restoration.

The long-term follow-up demonstrated excellent stability of esthetic peri-implant soft tissues for up to nine years. In particular, the facial mucosa maintained its convex contour and the height of the midfacial gingival margin without any recession (Figs 40 – 43).

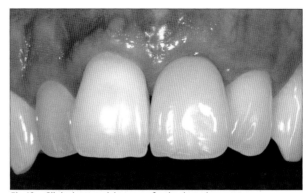

Fig 40   Clinical status eight years after implant placement.

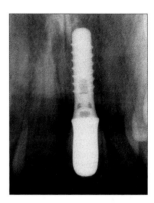

Fig 41   The radiographic follow-up at eight years showed excellent stability of the bone crest levels.

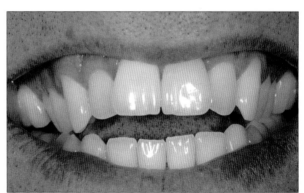

Fig 42   Clinical smile. The esthetic treatment outcome continues to be pleasing (December, 2005).

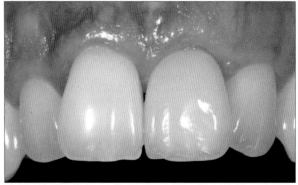

Fig 43   The detail view confirming the stability of the esthetic result at the nine-year follow-up.

4.2 Prosthetic Management of Implants in the Esthetic Zone: General Principles and Scientific Documentation

C. Hämmerle, R. Jung

When teeth in the esthetic zone are lost, implants often represent the therapy of choice. The patient will not only request restitution of health and function, but will also place strong emphasis on the esthetic outcome. In order to meet these expectations, the surgical and the prosthetic procedures need to be conducted using state-of-the-art methods and techniques. Because patients are interested in a pleasing appearance of their teeth and mucosa, surgical and prosthetic procedures need to be closely interlinked.

In recent years, there has been increasing evidence that a restoration-driven treatment concept is the key to achieving optimal outcomes in the esthetic zone.

What are the accepted criteria for considering a given treatment outcome an "esthetic success"? The third ITI Consensus Conference (Proceedings of the Third ITI Consensus Conference 2004) gave the following answer:

> **Statement C.1**
> **Standards for an Esthetic Fixed Implant Restoration**
> An esthetic implant prosthesis was defined as one that is in harmony with the perioral facial structures of the patient. The esthetic peri-implant tissues, including health, height, volume, color, and contours, must be in harmony with the healthy surrounding dentition. The restoration should imitate the natural appearance of the missing dental unit(s) in color, form, texture, size, and optical properties.

As stated by the third ITI Consensus Conference (Proceedings of the Third ITI Consensus Conference 2004) and illustrated in Chapter 3 and Section 4.1, proper patient selection, sound treatment planning, and correct three-dimensional implant placement following a restoration-driven approach are the basis for achieving esthetic treatment outcomes that remain stable over time.

> **Consensus Statement B.1**
> **Planning and Execution**
> Implant therapy in the anterior maxilla is considered an advanced or complex procedure and requires comprehensive preoperative planning and precise surgical execution based on a restoration-driven approach.

> **Consensus Statement B.2**
> **Patient Selection**
> Appropriate patient selection is essential in achieving esthetic treatment outcomes. Treatment of high-risk patients identified through site analysis and a general risk assessment (medical status, periodontal susceptibility, smoking, and other risks) should be undertaken with caution, since esthetic results are less consistent.

An important aspect of the prosthetic management of esthetic sites is related to the appropriate timing of implant loading. This is based on the fact that both the patient and the clinical team have a desire to reduce the overall treatment time.

The patient's individual risk profile as introduced in Chapter 3 of this book is the basis for the decision-making process in regard to the time of implant loading. It has to be kept in mind that the the primary objectives are to reach the treatment goals and to minimize the associated risk. Delayed loading (3 – 6 months after implantation) is therefore preferred in critical situations in order to minimize treatment risk. The topic of loading protocols in implant dentistry will be addressed in Volumes II and III of the ITI Treatment Guide and is not discussed in detail here.

The soft tissues around implant-supported prostheses are of primary importance for an esthetic treatment outcome. Esthetic peri-implant soft tissues are characterized by good tissue health and appropriate volume, color, and contours in harmony with the healthy surrounding tissues.

Keratinized peri-implant mucosa also integrates better with the surrounding structures than non-keratinized mucosa, from an esthetic point of view. The clinical team should therefore aim at establishing keratinized mucosa around a dental implant (Figs 1a-c; Alpert, 1994; Saadoun and coworkers, 1994; Landsberg, 1997; Jung and coworkers, 2004).

Multiple problems such as a lack of buccal soft-tissue height, a lack of papillary height, asymmetries, dislocation of the junction between attached and mobile mucosa, scars, irregular mucosal texture, and discolorations often pose obstacles to achieving optimal esthetics. Furthermore, clinically apparent ridge defects include underlying bony deficiencies in addition to soft-tissue deficits. As for the restorative aspects, three general levels can be identified that need to be taken into consideration in order to obtain an esthetically pleasing implant-supported restoration:

Level 1: Bone contour
Level 2: Soft-tissue contours and texture
Level 3: Prosthesis: contours, position, texture, and color

The underlying bone, the soft tissue, and the superstructure all affect the esthetic outcome. It is therefore recommended that the clinician move from one level to the next. Before or at implant placement, the bone contour is modified according to the existing functional and esthetic requirements. The soft-tissue management is carried out next, comprised of grafting with various techniques and of contouring with appropriate healing caps and provisional restorations. Finally, the prosthesis ("white esthetics") is fabricated.

Provided that the bone and soft tissue contours were preserved or appropriately optimized during pretreatment (Levels 1 and 2), ideal prerequisites are now established for the fabrication of an esthetic implant superstructure.

The soft-tissue contouring process is initiated before or at the time of implant site re-entry. Soft-tissue recession has to be expected within the first three to twelve months after abutment connection. In transmucosal healing, recession starts developing after implant insertion, whereas in submerged healing, this process begins only after abutment connection. On average, the amount of recession is between 0.6 and 1.6 mm, with considerable variation (Grunder, 2000; Oates and coworkers, 2002; Small and Tarnow, 2000; Ekfeldt and coworkers, 2003).

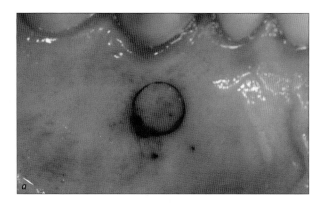
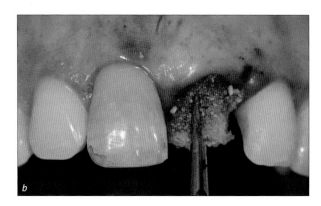
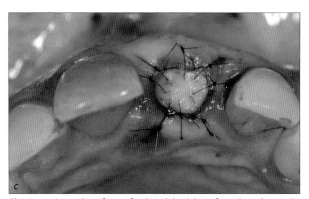

Figs 1a-c   A punch graft transfers keratinized tissue from the palate to the alveolus. A collagen allograft is used to fill the extraction socket for supporting the graft.

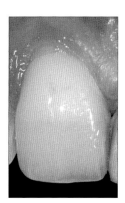

Fig 2   Thin, highly scalloped gingiva, combined with a soft-tissue and hard-tissue defect.

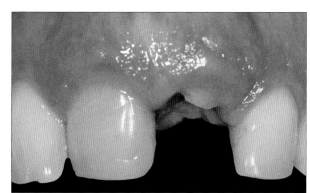

Fig 3   Soft-tissue access allowing for transmucosal healing.

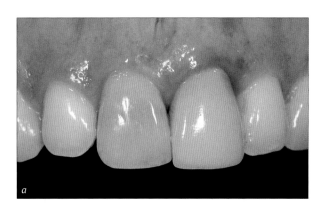

When it comes to deciding whether a submerged or a non-submerged approach is to be chosen, the following recommendations can be derived from the above literature:

1. In esthetically demanding areas with a thin, highly scalloped gingiva or where extensive soft-tissue or hard-tissue defects are present, submerged healing is recommended in order to establish soft-tissue access (Fig 2).
2. In esthetically demanding areas with a thick, low scalloped gingiva and soft-tissue access of at least 1 – 2 mm compared to the contralateral tooth, transmucosal healing can be chosen (Fig 3).

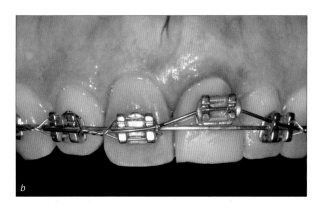

Statement B.5
Soft-Tissue Stability
For long-term esthetic soft-tissue stability, sufficient horizontal and vertical bone volume is essential. When deficiencies exist, appropriate hard and/or soft-tissue augmentation procedures are required. Currently, vertical bone deficiencies are a challenge to correct and often lead to esthetic shortcomings. To optimize soft-tissue volume, complete or partial coverage of the healing cap/implant is recommended in the anterior maxilla. In certain situations, a non-submerged approach can be considered.

Soft-tissue management can be carried out at different times relative to implant placement and abutment connection:

1. Before implant placement: in situations with extensive soft-tissue deficits (Figs 4a-c).
2. At implant placement with submerged healing: standard procedure for the correction of soft-tissue problems.

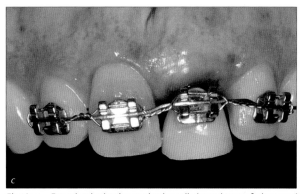

Figs 4a-c   Forced orthodontic eruption is applied to enlarge soft-tissue and hard-tissue volume.

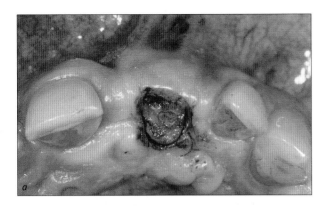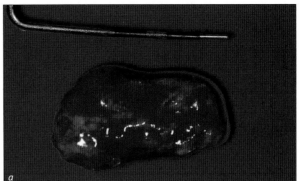

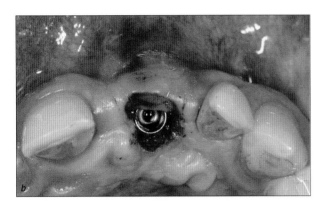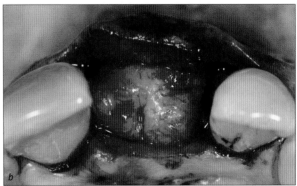

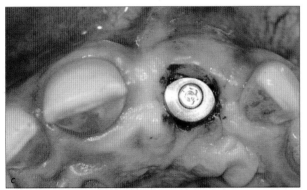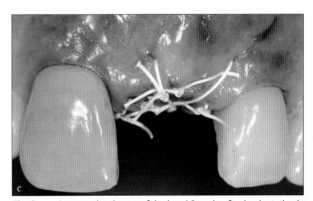

Figs 5a-c   A semilunar incision and subsequent rolling of a de-epithelial-ized pedicle flap in a buccal direction. Tissue loss is avoided and the labial soft-tissue contour is improved.

Figs 6a-c   A connective tissue graft is placed 6 weeks after implantation in order to improve the soft-tissue contours.

3. At abutment connection with submerged healing or at implant placement with transmucosal healing (for the correction of minor soft-tissue problems only) (Figs 5a-c).
4. After placement of a temporary or final reconstruction (in exceptional cases only).

Soft-tissue corrections before implant insertion may be necessary in rare cases to allow secure implantation, whereas additional soft tissue can more easily be incorporated directly at the time of implantation. In the majority of cases, soft-tissue corrections are performed after implant placement, since the exact implant position and the amount of augmented bone are only clear at this time (Figs 6a-c).

Soft-tissue defects that remain after implant placement are corrected before or at the time of healing cap/abutment connection.

Earlier protocols for abutment connection describe a punch technique under local anesthesia to gain access to the implant shoulder (Lekholm, 1983). This excision technique does not consider factors such as the mucosal thickness, the soft-tissue profile, or the course of the transition line between keratinized and non-keratinized mucosa. In addition, precious soft tissue is sacrificed by this technique. In order to maintain as much tissue as possible and to minimize the risks, resection techniques are usually avoided.

The following overview of implant exposure (reentry) techniques for abutment connection can be given:

- Punch technique (only where abundant volume and width of keratinized mucosa are present)
- Crestal or paracrestal incision of the keratinized mucosa with apical positioning of the vestibular mucosa
- Roll technique utilizing mini-flaps

The reentry procedure can also be considered an opportunity to influence the keratinized mucosa with respect to contour and volume by applying reconstructive techniques. Accordingly, reentry does not merely serve the purpose of uncovering the implant and choosing appropriate healing caps, but it is also an opportunity for establishing of functional and esthetic peri-implant soft tissue.

During the subsequent wound healing and soft-tissue maturation period, the new soft-tissue situation is supported and stabilized by the healing cap and the provisional crown. It is important to note that there are very few chances left to manipulate the soft-tissue contours after the insertion of the provisional or the final crown. At that stage, vertical augmentation is no longer possible. A deficient slight soft-tissue volume can be remedied using inlay-grafting techniques (Fig 5). Hence, it is important to anticipate soft-tissue problems before the insertion of healing caps or provisionals. There are hardly any options for corrections after that point.

Bearing the above in mind, the aims of the abutment-connection procedure can be summarized as follows:

In traditional implant dentistry:

- Creation of a connection of the dental implant to the oral cavity

In esthetic implant dentistry additionally:

- Assessment of the bone volume surrounding the implant after guided bone regeneration (GBR) procedures and, if required, membrane removal
- Widening of the band of keratinized mucosa
- Relocation of the mucogingival border
- Enlargement of the volume of the buccal/labial mucosa in order to improve the ridge contour (root prominence)
- Augmentation of interproximal soft tissues for papilla reconstruction

The circular profile of most healing caps differs from the rather triangular profile of the cervical portion of the tooth to be reconstructed. Hence, adjustments in shape need to be made in order to create a natural, esthetic emergence profile. This can best be achieved by temporary crowns or by the final restoration with the desired shape and contour.

From a biological point of view and with regard to tissue stability over time, a provisional crown is not mandatory. This assertion is based on the observation that the papillae adjacent to single-implant restorations present similar volume two years after crown insertion, regardless of the types of the abutments used (healing cap or provisional resin crown; Jemt and coworkers, 1999). The same study also demonstrated that the shape of the peri-implant soft tissues was achieved more quickly using provisional crowns than with healing caps.

Consensus Statement C.4
Use of Provisional Restorations
To optimize esthetic treatment outcomes, the use of provisional restorations with adequate emergence profiles is recommended to guide and shape the peri-implant tissue before definitive restoration.

In addition, temporary crowns are also valuable in diagnostics with regard to the (future) peri-implant soft-tissue esthetics as well as to the ideal shape of the final crown. Therefore, it is highly recommended to use provisional crowns in esthetic sites.

It can be advantageous to adapt the shape of the provisional crown at chairside. This allows the establishment of the ideal shape, size, and contour in a single step or in multiple steps. This can be done by subtracting (Paul and Jovanovic 1999) or by adding temporary material (Figs 7 a, b). Depending on the desired emergence profile and the quality of the mucosa, one to three conditioning steps, i.e. modifications of the shape of the crown, are necessary (Touati, 1995; Potashnick, 1998; Vogel, 2002). Within six to eight weeks, this process leads to the final soft-tissue contour (Hinds, 1997; Vogel, 2002).

Maturation and stabilization of the peri-implant mucosa around a provisional crown take place within the first three to twelve months after insertion (Grunder, 2000; Oates and coworkers, 2002; Small and Tarnow, 2000; Ekfeldt and coworkers, 2003). It is therefore recommended that the provisional crown remain in situ for at least three months.

When the desired shape and emergence profile are achieved (Fig 8), the impression for the master cast and the final crown fabrication is taken.

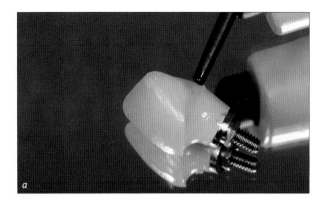

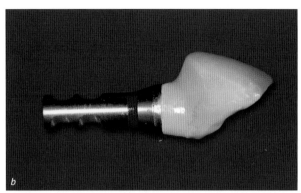

Figs 7a, b   The cervical portion of the provisional crown is reshaped at chairside.

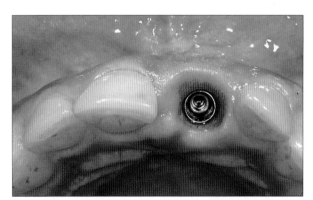

Fig 8   The contours of the mucosa for a natural emergence profile, which were shaped by the provisional, can now be captured with the impression.

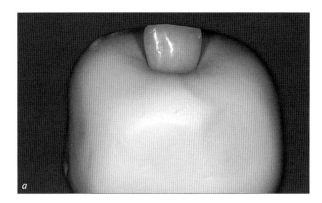

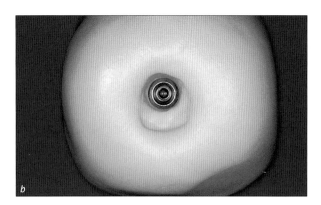

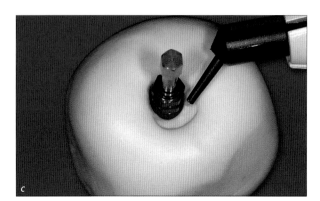

A so-called individualized impression that transfers the emergence profile by use of an impression cap is advantageous in esthetic sites (Figs 9a-d).

It precisely captures the emergence profile of the final provisional crown and thus accurately communicates the desired clinical situation to the dental technician (Figs 10 a – b).

In the following situations, the use of a provisional crown is highly recommended:

1. Patient has high expectations regarding the esthetic treatment outcome and/or optimal esthetics
2. Patient presents thin, highly scalloped gingival biotype
3. Need for additional diagnostics regarding the shape or position of the planned reconstruction

In summary, the timing of the soft-tissue conditioning process from the first impression to incorporation of the final crown is as follows (Fig 11):

The transition zone, i.e., the emergence profile created from the shoulder of the implant to the soft-tissue margin, can either be conditioned by a transocclusally screw-retained crown (provisional or final) or by a mesostructure such as the synOcta gold abutment or the synOcta In-Ceram blank. A mesostructure may be beneficial whenever access to the implant shoulder is difficult to obtain. This is frequently the case in the interproximal areas of the esthetic zone, where the implant shoulder can easily be located 5 or even 6 mm submucosally.

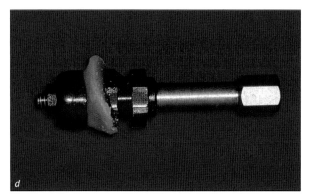

Figs 9a-d   An extraoral impression of the provisional crown is used to transfer the desired emergence profile to the impression cap.

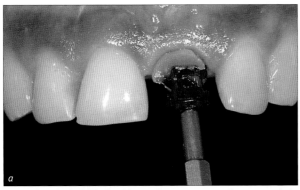
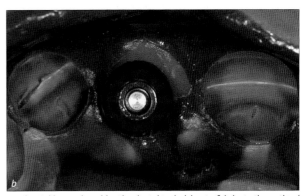

Fig 10a-b   The individualized impression cap supports the mucosa during impression taking and enables the dental technician to fabricate the optimal shape of the final crown.

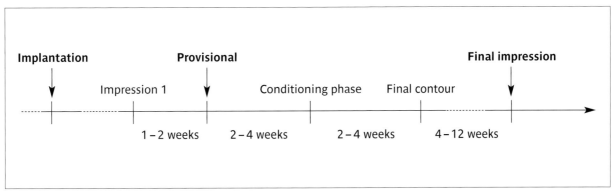

Fig 11   Timing of the soft-tissue conditioning process in esthetic sites.

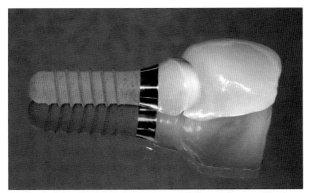

Fig 12   Individualized zirconia abutment and all-ceramic crown. The shape of the crown margin is favorable, facilitating effective cement removal.

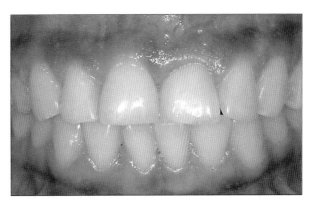

Fig 13   After adhesive cementation of the all-ceramic crown 21, harmonious integration into the natural dentition could be observed.

A mesostructure, i.e., an individualized abutment, not only serves to condition the mucosa in the transition zone, but it also displaces the margin of the crown coronally (Fig 12). Thus, the margin of the crown is located closer to the soft-tissue margin for better access to effectively remove the cement used for seating crown (Higginbottom and coworkers, 2004). Furthermore, a mesostructure may help compensate for a non-ideal implant axis.

When a mesostructure is used, it is recommendable to try in this mesostructure in order to optimize the position and shape of the future crown margin (Fig 13). This ensures pleasing esthetics and facilitates thorough cement removal.

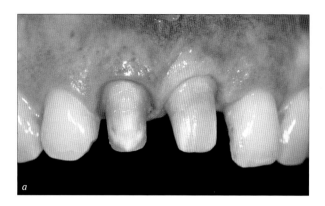

The biocompatibility of the various abutment materials used also plays an important role. Commercially pure titanium as well as aluminum oxide and zirconia ceramics are the abutment materials of choice (Figs 14a-c).

An epithelial attachment has been shown to form on these materials, resulting in stable peri-implant tissue.

By contrast, soft-tissue recession and cervical bone resorption have been found with gold and ceramic veneer (Abrahamsson and coworkers, 1998; Kohal, 2004).

Another important aspect is the mechanical properties of the materials. High-strength ceramic materials such as densely sintered aluminum oxide or zirconia exhibit fracture resistance values high enough for these materials to be used intraorally (Lüthy, 1996; Seghi and coworkers, 1995).

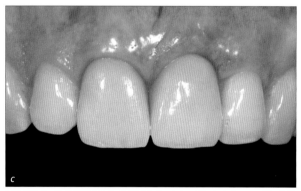

The thickness of the peri-implant mucosa is also a critical factor for the selection of the appropriate abutment material. In situations where the thickness was larger than 2.5 mm, the color of the abutment did not negatively influence the color of the mucosa (Hämmerle and coworkers, 2005). It may be be surmised that in esthetically demanding locations in combination with a mucosal thickness below 2.5 mm, ceramic abutments avoid possible negative influences on the esthetic treatment outcome. Further research, however, is required before clear-cut clinical recommendations can be made.

Figs 14a-c   In-Ceram blank at site 21, frontal and incisal view, and final situation with all-ceramic crown on tooth 11 and all-ceramic implant-supported superstructure at site 21.

Acknowledgment

The authors express their special thanks to master dental technician Ana Suter for her expert technical work presented in this chapter.

4.3 Decision Trees: Prosthetic Options

U. C. Belser

The decision trees* for Regular Neck (RN) and Narrow Neck (NN) implants presented in this chapter were developed to illustrate, in a structured manner, the possible prosthetic options available in a given clinical situation once the implant has been inserted. In this context, the specific design of both the provisional crown and the final superstructure, whether screw-retained or cemented, and their respective restorative components (abutments, mesostructures, secondary and tertiary components) are graphically presented.

The different prosthetic options suggested in the decision trees relate primarily to the individual implant position, which includes both implantation depth as well as implant axis.

The options suggested reflect the recommendations of the third consensus conference (group on esthetics) and do not claim to be "general rules."

The decision trees are not meant to provide a complete list of all available restorative components of the Straumann Dental Implant System, nor do they represent a definite hierarchy of prosthetic options. They reflect the authors' personal opinion, which is based on clinical experience.

The options based on ceramics (whether screw-retained or cemented) were listed as the first options in order to take into account the most recent developments in anterior implant prosthodontics (CAD/CAM technology, ZrO_2). This does not put ceramo-metal restorations in the position of "second choice" by any means.

Blank fields for specific combinations of implant depths and orofacial implant axes represent theoretical options for superstructures that, in the opinion of the authors, are less recommendable, even if they are theoretically possible.

Since the rational choice of the most appropriate material (titanium/gold alloys/ceramics) in a specific given situation was discussed in detail in section 4.2 "Prosthetic Management of Implants in the Esthetic Zone," this discussion will not be revisited in this section.

4.3.1 Regular Neck Implants

The Regular Neck implant decision tree* is structured in matrix form. The top row represents, from left to right, the three possible vertical implant shoulder positions (i.e., ideal, deep, superficial) and secondly an axial-position problem. By definition, this last aspect can be "superimposed" on any of the three preceding situations. The columns reflect the possible restorative options relative to implant shoulder depth and implant axis, in the following order:

- Provisional implant restorations (screw-retained/cemented)
- Definitive implant restorations
    - All-ceramic restorations, screw-retained
    - All-ceramic restorations, cemented
    - Ceramo-metal restorations, screw-retained
    - Ceramo-metal restorations, cemented

We deliberately limited this decision tree to the two variables "implantation depth" and "orofacial axial-position problem," because we consider that the remainder of theoretically possible implant positioning „errors" such as:

- Position too far mesial/distal
- Position too far labial/palatal
- Axial-position problem in the frontal plane

These errors should not occur under normal conditions.

As mentioned above, certain fields were left blank, indicating this that specific restorative option cannot be recommended, given the particular implant-shoulder depth or orofacial axial-position problem:

* For the decision-tree posters, please see the inside back cover.

Row 3: In case of a significantly protruding implant axis, a transocclusally screw-retained all-ceramic solution is literally impossible.

Row 4: In case of a superficial implant shoulder position, an all-ceramic restoration cemented on a CARES custom abutment cannot be recommended, as the respective cemented interface would be located too close to the labial mucosal margin.

Rows 5, 6, and 7: In case of a superficial implant-shoulder position or an orofacial axial-position problem, a transocclusally screw-retained ceramo-metal restoration cannot be recommended, as the metal margin would be too close to the mucosal margin and the screw access channel would be located on the labial aspect of the restoration.

Rows 8 and 14: In the absence of an orofacial axial-position problem, the use of an angulated abutment does not make sense.

Rows 9 and 10: In case of a deep or a superficial implant shoulder position, a transversally screw-retained restoration is not recommended, as in the first case the screw-access channel may be located submucosally, and in the second case, this same screw-access channel may interfere with the occlusion.

Rows 11 and 12: In case of a superficial implant shoulder position, the use of a CARES titanium custom abutment or a synOcta gold abutment as a mesostructure for a cemented ceramo-metal restoration is not recommended, as the cemented interface would be too close to the labial mucosal margin.

Row 13: In case of an ideal or a deep implant shoulder position, a ceramo-metal restoration cemented on a prefabricated solid abutment cannot be recommended, as the interproximal crown margins are inaccessible and the resulting cement excess is difficult to remove.

It should generally be noted, however, that a ceramo-metal implant shoulder is theoretically also possible in case of a superficial implant shoulder position (although the respective column was deliberately left blank), provided the dental technician has the requisite know-how and skills to produce a metal margin of only minimal width (no more than 0.2 – 0.4 mm). If this is an option, visible metal margins can usually be avoided.

4.3.2 Narrow Neck Implants

The Narrow Neck implant decision tree* has also been structured in the form of a matrix. The top row represents, from left to right, first the three possible vertical implant shoulder positions – ideal, deep, superficial – and secondly an axial-position problem in orofacial direction. As per definition, this last aspect can be "superimposed" on any of the three preceding situations. The vertical columns reflect the possible restorative options relative to implant shoulder sink depth and implant axis, in the following order:

- Provisional implant restorations
  (screw-retained/cemented)
- Definitive implant restorations
    - Ceramo-metal restorations, screw-retained
    - Ceramo-metal restorations, cemented

A ceramic abutment (ZrO_2) for use with Straumann CARES, the Computer Aided REstoration Service, will be available in 2007.

We have deliberately limited this decision tree to the two variables "implantation depth" and "orofacial axial-position problem," as we consider that the remainder of the theoretically possible implant positioning "errors" should not occur under normal conditions:

- Position too far mesial/distal
- Position too far labial/palatal
- Axial-position problem in the frontal plane

As mentioned above, certain fields have been left blank, indicating that this specific restorative option cannot be recommended, given the particular implant shoulder depth or orofacial axial-position problem:

Rows 4 and 5: In case of a significant orofacial axial-position problem, a transocclusally screw-retained ceramo-metal restoration cannot be recommended, as the screw-access channel would be located on the labial aspect of the restoration.

Rows 6 and 8: In case of a superficial implant shoulder position or an orofacial axial-position problem, a cemented ceramo-metal restoration cannot be recommended, as in the first case the cemented interface lies too close to the soft-tissue margin, and in the second case the underlying abutment would not provide adequate retention/resistance form after having corrected the axial-position problem.

Row 7: In the absence of an orofacial axial-position problem, the use of an angulated abutment does not make sense.

4.4 Replacement of an Upper Right Central Incisor with a Regular Neck Implant, Restored with an All-Ceramic Crown, Transocclusally Screw-Retained

R. Jung

This 37-year-old female patient, a non-smoker, complained about discomfort and gingival problems at tooth 11. She was in good general health, and her medical history was without significant findings.

The clinical inspection of the oral cavity revealed a fistula originating at tooth 11 (Fig 1).

Radiological examination of the crowned tooth 11 revealed a root-canal filling, status after apicoectomy, and a large periapical bone defect, as well as secondary caries (Fig 2).

The adjacent teeth, 21 and 12, were periodontally healthy. They had interdental composite fillings that the patient wanted replaced. The bone crest levels of teeth 12 and 21 were well maintained, providing potential soft-tissue support (Fig 3).

The treatment approach would have to ensure that the distance between the interproximal bone crests of the neighboring teeth and the contact with the planned implant-supported superstructure would not exceed 5 mm, as this has been proven to be an important factor for the predictability of the papillae (Tarnow and coworkers, 1992).

Periodontal probing of tooth 11 as well as teeth 12 and 21 showed probing depths not exceeding 4 mm.

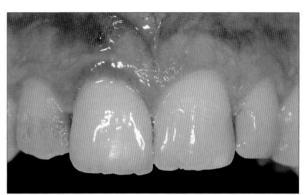

Fig 1   The fistula buccally of tooth 11 is clearly visible.

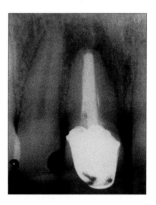

Fig 2   Radiograph of tooth 11 with periapical pathology.

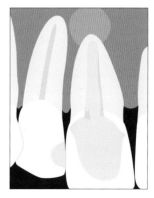

Fig 3   The interproximal bone levels are intact. Because of the large periapical radiolucency, however, an extensive bone defect had to be anticipated.

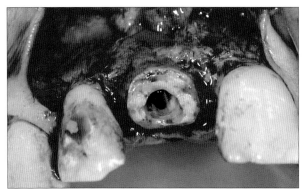

Fig 4   A bony defect was to be expected despite the harmoniously contoured bony arch.

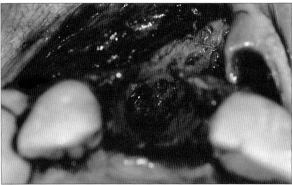

Fig 5   Buccal view of the treatment site after a mucoperiosteal flap was raised. Note the lack of labial bone around the root to be extracted.

Fig 6   After the extraction and removal of the granulation tissue, a large bone defect was present that did not allow for primary implant stability.

The patient's biotype was medium thick, with a medium scallop height. The soft tissues were free of recessions and other defects. The gingival margin of contralateral tooth 21 was located about 1 mm further apically than that of tooth 11, so there was some "soft-tissue access." The shape of the tooth crown was rectangular. The shape of the gingival margin was harmonious, as was the shape of the incisal edges, except for the elongated crown of tooth 11.

Clinically, the bony arch presented harmonious contours, but due to the large periapical radiolucency, a bony defect had to be anticipated (Fig 4).

The clinical and radiological findings in this patient add up to the following esthetic risk-profile analysis (Table 1):

The individual esthetic risk profile of this patient shows that this case is to be considered a medium-risk case. This means that a certain esthetic risk is associated with the treatment of this patient concerning the esthetic treatment outcome.

Based upon the clinical and radiological findings and the assessment of the esthetic risk associated with the treatment, a treatment plan was defined with a two-stage treatment protocol, including a guided bone-regeneration procedure and the placement of a Straumann Standard Plus dental implant at site 11.

A full-thickness flap was raised for tooth extraction and bone augmentation. Tooth 11 was extracted (Figs 5, 6).

Table 1 The patient's individual esthetic risk profile.

Esthetic Risk Factors	Low	Medium	High
Medical status	Healthy patient and intact immune system		Reduced immune system
Smoking habit	Non-smoker	Light smoker (< 10 cig/d)	Heavy smoker (> 10 cig/d)
Patient's esthetic expectations	Low	Medium	High
Lip line	Low	Medium	High
Gingival biotype	Low scalloped, thick	Medium scalloped, medium thick	High scalloped, thin
Shape of tooth crowns	Rectangular	Slightly triangular	Triangular
Infection at implant site	None	Chronic	Acute
Bone level at adjacent teeth	≤ 5 mm to contact point	5.5 to 6.5 mm to contact point	≥ 7 mm to contact point
Restorative status of neighboring teeth	Virgin		Restored
Width of edentulous span	1 tooth (≥ 7 mm)	1 tooth (< 7 mm)	2 teeth or more
Soft-tissue anatomy	Intact soft tissue		Soft-tissue defects
Bone anatomy of alveolar crest	Alveolar crest without bone deficiency	Horizontal bone deficiency	Vertical bone deficiency

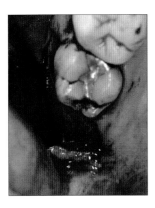

Fig 7   Access to the donor site at the tuberosity area was gained with horizontal (tuber), vertical (mesial to tooth 17), and sulcular (tooth 17) incisions and mucoperiosteal flap elevation.

A large bone defect was present after the extraction and removal of the granulation tissue. Due to the severe bone resorption caused by the infection, a bone-augmentation procedure needed to be performed before implant insertion (Fig 6). Thanks to the favorable anatomy of the defect and the protective walls of the extraction socket, a bone-augmentation procedure with particulate grafting material and a resorbable membrane was chosen.

Autogenous bone was harvested from the tuberosity area of the left upper quadrant using forceps and chisels (Figs 7, 8). Access to that area is similar to the procedure for extracting a third molar.

The autogenous bone was then applied to the alveolus and subsequently covered with a layer of deproteinized bovine bone mineral (DBBM) (Fig 9).

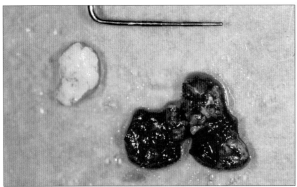

Fig 8   Particulate autogenous bone harvested form the tuberosity area.

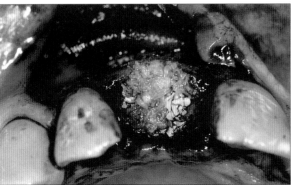

Fig 9   Alveolar defect filled up using the GBR technique and autogenous bone and particles of DBBM as supporting material.

The augmentation site was then covered with a collagen membrane (Figs 9, 10).

The augmented area was carefully shaped to the desired contour. The labial aspect of the future implant site was slightly overcontoured to create a favorable bone volume and shape (Fig 11).

To facilitate primary wound closure without advancing the buccal flap too far coronally, a rotational pedicle graft was prepared (Fig 12) and rotated over the grafted alveolar region (Fig 13). The graft was prepared by splitting the palatal flap from the distal to the mesial end and leaving the pedicle at the site of the former extraction socket.

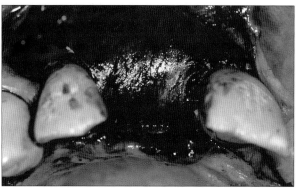

Fig 10   The augmented area was covered with a resorbable collagen membrane stabilized with two resorbable pins in the apical region. Note the overcontoured labial aspect of the prospective implant site.

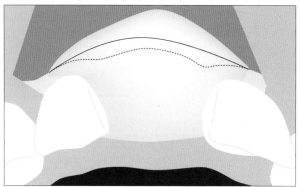

Fig 11   About one-fourth of the volume was overcontoured in order to compensate for the volume reduction caused by soft-tissue pressure.

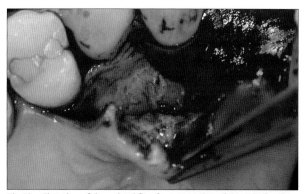

Fig 12   Elevation of the palatal flap for preparation of the split flap from distal to mesial.

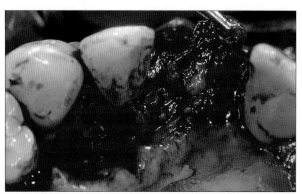

Fig 13   Elevation of the connective-tissue pedicle graft to the site of augmentation.

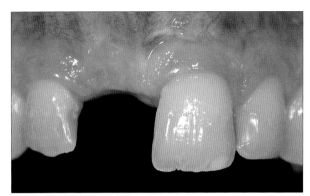

Fig 14   Site 11 six months after primary augmentation.

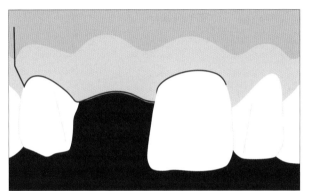

Fig 15   Incision technique: sulcular incision around teeth 12 and 21; crestal incision slightly palatally; vertical releasing incision distally of tooth 12.

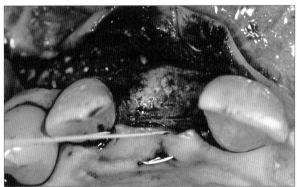

Fig 16   Occlusal view of the regenerated augmented bone area.

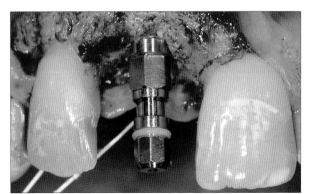

Fig 17   Implant in the correct vertical position.

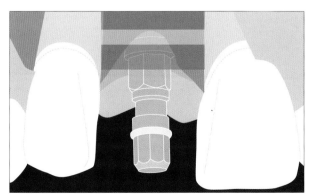

Fig 18   The implant shoulder was located in the coronoapical comfort zone.

Six months after augmentation, the site was healthy and stable (Fig 14) and could be reopened for implant placement.

To ensure good blood supply and to minimize the trauma to the soft tissue, only one vertical relieving incision was made (Fig 15).

As the full-thickness flap was created, care was taken to place the crestal incision slightly palatally to avoid cutting through the tip of the papilla.

Bone volume and contour proved to be favorable as the flap was elevated. The new bone was vital and well supplied with blood. Note the slightly overcontoured bone at the facial aspect (Fig 16).

A Standard Plus implant was then placed in an ideal three-dimensional position (Figs 17, 19).

In the coronoapical dimension, care was taken to place the implant shoulder approximately 1 mm apically of the cemento-enamel junction of contralateral tooth 21 (Figs 17, 18).

Also in the orofacial dimension, the implant shoulder was placed in an ideal position, i.e. about 1 mm palatally of the point of emergence of the adjacent teeth (Figs 19, 20). Note the remaining thickness of the facial bone wall of more than 1 mm.

The implant was covered with a closure screw. The flap was sutured for the implant to osseointegrate in a sub-merged healing mode. The flap was sutured with non-re-sorbable ePTFE suture material.

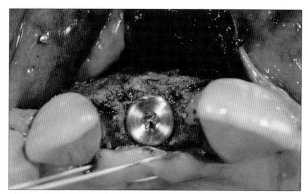

Fig 19   Occlusal view of the correct orofacial position of the implant.

Twelve weeks after implant placement, the closure screw was replaced by a labially beveled healing cap in order to start the mucosa-conditioning phase and to facilitate soft-tissue contouring. Two weeks later, remarkably good soft-tissue access was seen at the facial aspect of the implant site. An impression was taken for a provisional crown (Fig 22).

Four months after the implant was placed, a temporary crown with a moderate emergence profile was fabricated by the dental technician using a titanium post for tempo-rary restorations (Fig 23). At the time of integration of the temporary crown, it is important not to put too much pressure on the soft tissue. Instead, the emergence pro-file should be moderate, so that it can be modified in one or two subsequent steps. This step-by-step procedure pre-vents soft-tissue retraction and helps build a perfectly conditioned mucosa to match the emergence line and the contour of the marginal gingiva of the contralateral tooth as closely as possible.

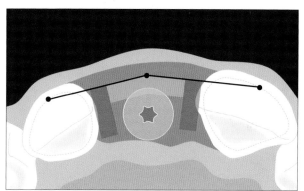

Fig 20   The implant shoulder was located in the orofacial comfort zone.

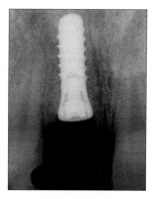

Fig 21   Radiograph of the inserted implant during submerged healing.

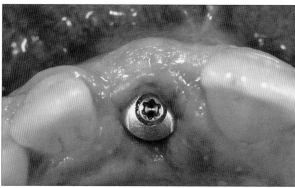

Fig 22   Clinical situation two weeks after abutment insertion.

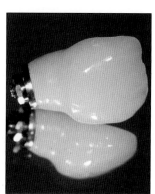

Fig 23   Temporary crown with mod-erate emergence profile.

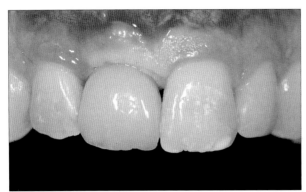

Fig 24 The pressure of the inserted temporary crown caused soft-tissue blanching.

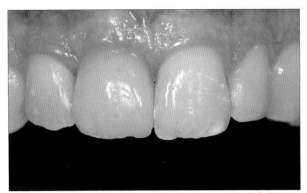

Fig 25 Emergence profile of the provisional as improved by chairside step-by-step modification with light-curing composite.

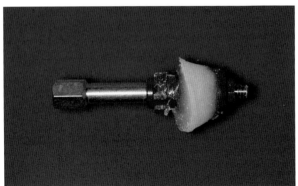

Fig 26 Modified impression cap capturing the shape of the provisional crown.

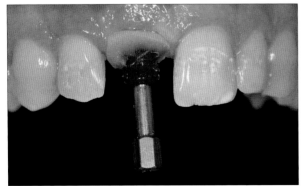

Fig 27 Modified impression coping in place.

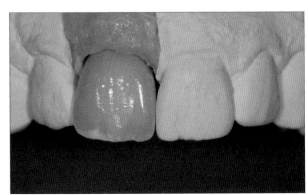

Fig 28 Frontal view of the all-ceramic crown (synOcta In-Ceram blank).

The clinical situation immediately after insertion of the temporary crown showed soft-tissue blanching caused by pressure (Fig 24). The temporary crown did not yet have the desired shape, and the line of emergence did not yet match that of the contralateral tooth 21.

In order to improve the shape and emergence profile, the provisional was modified chairside with a light curing composite material (Fig 25).

After a soft-tissue maturation phase of three months, a custom impression cap was produced, capturing the shape of the provisional crown's cervical portion and transferring it to the prefabricated impression cap (Fig 26).

At impression-taking, this customized impression coping prevented soft-tissue collapse and ensured optimal support of the emergence profile (Fig 27).

The final crown was fabricated at the dental laboratory using a synOcta In-Ceram blank (Fig 28).

Thanks to the ideal implant axis, a screw-retained crown could be fabricated (Fig 29).

For crown fabrication, the In-Ceram blank was ground to the shape of a miniature copy of tooth 11, which was subsequently glass-infiltrated and directly veneered with a veneering ceramic.

The screw head was sealed off with a thin layer of cotton, and the screw access was finally closed off with a light-curing composite material. The occlusion was carefully checked.

The screw-retained all-ceramic crown harmoniously integrated into the row of natural teeth. Another very important advantage of screw retention was that there was no cement residue after crown cementation (Fig 30).

The 2.5-year follow-up photograph confirmed stable peri-implant soft tissues (Fig 31).

The 2.5-year follow-up periapical radiograph confirmed stable peri-implant bone levels (Fig 32).

Acknowledgments

Prosthetic Procedures
Dr. David Siegenthaler – University of Zurich, Switzerland, Clinic for Dental Crown and Bridge Prosthetics, Partial Prosthetics, and Dental Material Science

Dr. Claudia Holderegger – University of Zurich, Switzerland, Clinic for Dental Crown and Bridge Prosthetics, Partial Prosthetics, and Dental Material Science

Laboratory Procedures
Master Dental Technician Ana Suter – University of Zurich, Switzerland, Clinic for Dental Crown and Bridge Prosthetics, Partial Prosthetics, and Dental Material Science

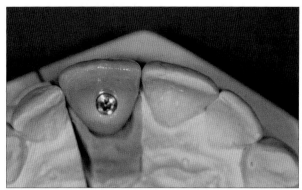

Fig 29   Occlusal view of the screw-retained all-ceramic crown (synOcta In-Ceram blank).

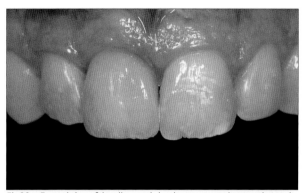

Fig 30   Frontal view of the all-ceramic implant-supported restoration at site 11.

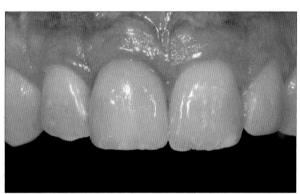

Fig 31   Clinical situation showing favorable soft-tissue contours 2.5 years after crown insertion.

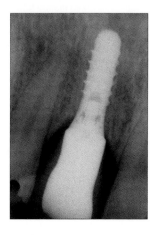

Fig 32   Stable peri-implant bone levels 2.5 years after crown insertion.

4.5 Replacement of an Upper Right Central Incisor with a Regular Neck Implant, Restored with (1) an All-Ceramic Crown, Transocclusally Screw-Retained, and (2) an Auro-Galvano Crown, Cemented, Seated on CAD/CAM Custom Mesostructures (ZrO$_2$ and Titanium)

U. C. Belser

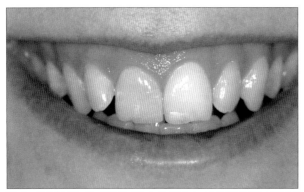

Fig 1   At full smile, the high lip line completely exposed the facial aspect of the anterior maxillary dentition, including the associated gingiva.

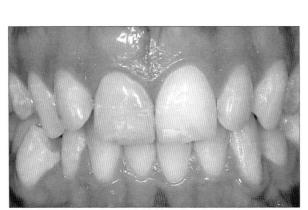

Fig 2   The thin to medium-thick, highly scalloped tissue biotype increased the overall esthetic risk in this patient.

In February 2005, a 25-year-old female patient, a non-smoker, was referred to our clinic due to tooth 11 presenting a chronic fistula following unsuccessful root-canal treatment and several attempts at endodontic surgery. The dental history revealed that more than ten years earlier, teeth 11 and 21 had been traumatized during a sports accident. Consequently, 11 had lost its vitality, and there were two moderate fractures of the mesioincisal borders of the two central incisors that had been restored with direct composite restorations.

At the time of examination, the composite restorations showed signs of wear, some discoloration, and marginal infiltration. The patient also complained about a moderate discoloration of the clinical crown of the non-vital tooth 11.

The patient was in good general health, and her medical history revealed no significant findings.

Tooth 11 was considered hopeless (irrational to treat), and implant therapy was the first therapeutic choice, as the neighboring teeth did not require significant restorations.

At full smile, the patient presented a high lip-line situation, completely exposing the anterior maxillary teeth and the associated facial gingival tissue (Fig 1).

The patient's gingival biotype was thin to medium thick and highly scalloped, at the same time presenting a broad band of keratinized mucosa (Fig 2).

The clinical examination revealed the presence of a chronic fistula apically of tooth 11 (Fig 3).

The initial radiographic examination documented a status after extensive conventional root-canal treatment followed by an unsuccessful attempt at periapical endodontic therapy, as well as pronounced apical and lateral root resorption. The vertical level of the interproximal bone at the adjacent teeth, however, was still within the physiological distance from the respective cemento-enamel junction (CEJ) of the adjacent teeth. This parameter represents a major prognostic factor for esthetic considerations relative to anterior single-tooth implant therapy (Fig 4).

The patient's subjective symptoms at site 11, with chronic pain and a persisting active fistula, and the highly unfavorable radiographic status made it irrational to try to re-treat this tooth. After a comprehensive evaluation of the various treatment options, single-tooth implant therapy was chosen, as it represented the least invasive treatment modality, preserving hard tissue at adjacent teeth, an approach that was highly predictable, also with regard to long-term esthetics (Belser and coworkers, 2003; Belser and coworkers, 2004; Buser and coworkers, 2004; Higginbottom and coworkers, 2004).

The above findings led to the following esthetic profile (Table 1), which could be classified as medium to high and was thus associated with a considerable esthetic risk:

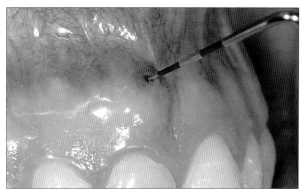

Fig 3   Periodontal probe, confirming the presence of a chronic fistula at the mucogingival border labial of root 11.

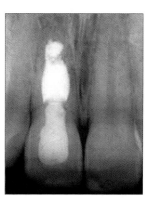

Fig 4   Initial periapical radiograph. Status after extensive conventional root-canal therapy on tooth 11, including an unsuccessful attempt at periapical endodontic surgery. Advanced apical and lateral root resorption. The vertical bone height at adjacent teeth was within two millimeters of the cemento-enamel junction.

Table 1 The patient's individual esthetic risk profile

Esthetic Risk Factors	Low	Medium	High
Medical status	Healthy and cooperative patient and intact immune system		Reduced immune system
Smoking habit	Non-smoker	Light smoker (< 10 cig/d)	Heavy smoker (> 10 cig/d)
Patient's esthetic expectations	Low	Medium	High
Lip line	Low	Medium	High
Gingival biotype	Low scalloped, thick	Medium scalloped, medium thick	High scalloped, thin
Shape of tooth crowns	Rectangular		Triangular
Infection at implant site	None	Chronic	Acute
Bone level at adjacent teeth	≤ 5 mm to contact point	5.5 to 6.5 mm to contact point	≥ 7 mm to contact point
Restorative status of neighboring teeth	21: minimally restored 12: virgin		Restored
Width of edentulous span	1 tooth (≥ 7 mm)	1 tooth (< 7 mm)	2 teeth or more
Soft-tissue anatomy	Intact soft tissue		Soft-tissue defects
Bone anatomy of alveolar crest	Alveolar crest without bone deficiency	Horizontal bone deficiency	Vertical bone deficiency

After careful analysis of the patient's esthetic risk profile, it was decided to proceed according to the well-documented early implant placement/early implant loading protocol, which implies a soft-tissue healing period of six to eight weeks after tooth extraction.

A simple partial denture was therefore fabricated to serve as an interim restoration during the first healing period (after tooth extraction) and the second healing period (after implant placement) (Fig 5).

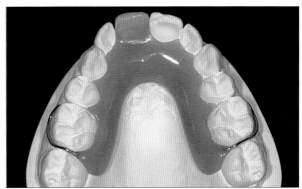

Fig 5 Occlusal view of the maxillary study cast with the simple removable partial denture, which was to serve as an interim restoration after the extraction of tooth 11.

With the tooth to be extracted still in place, the laboratory technician precisely anticipated on the study cast the local site configuration expected after tooth removal. In this process, the tooth was hemisected exactly at the gingival level. A discrete concavity was created at the same site in order to adapt a prefabricated acrylic denture tooth as an ovate pontic. The landmarks provided by the contralateral tooth helped create a simple but esthetically pleasing provisional that did not have a buccal denture flange, as no soft-tissue deficiencies had to be compensated for at this stage of treatment (Fig 6).

During the second appointment, tooth 11 was carefully and gently extracted without elevating a flap, using small desmotomes. Particular care was taken to avoid any mobilization of the root in a vestibular direction in order to preserve as much of the remaining buccal bone plate as possible (Fig 7).

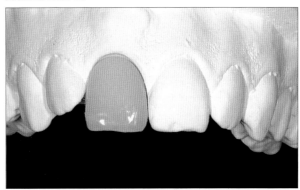

Fig 6 Labial aspect of the provisional removable partial denture (RPD). The laboratory technician had tried to respect, as much as possible, the symmetry-related esthetic parameters gathered from the contralateral site (21). In particular, the cervical aspect of temporary tooth 11 had been designed as an ovate pontic of a conventional fixed partial denture (FPD) without a labial denture flange.

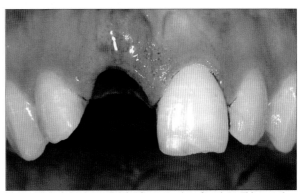

Fig 7 Clinical view immediately after extraction of tooth 11. This procedure was performed without elevating a mucoperiosteal flap.

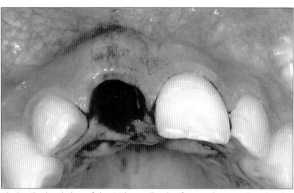

Fig 8   Occlusal view of site 11 immediately after tooth extraction showing the amount and extent of the vestibular soft-tissue swelling due to the active periapical inflammatory process.

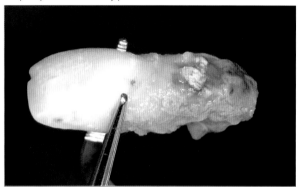

Fig 9   Examination of the extracted root. Mid-facial perforation, periapical root resorption, and abundant inflammatory tissue.

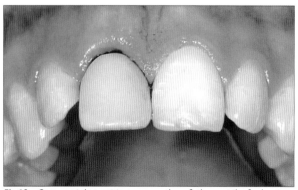

Fig 10   Care was taken not to compress the soft tissue at the fresh extraction site with the removable provisional partial denture, while also providing minimal tissue support in the interproximal areas.

The presence of an active periapical inflammatory process with associated pain, swelling (Fig 8), and a persisting fistula was incompatible with a more progressive and more rapid approach, such as the immediate placement of an implant.

Once the infected tooth 11 had been removed, the significant root resorption and abundant presence of granulation tissue fully confirmed the indication for an extraction (Fig 9).

Following the extraction, the previously fabricated provisional RPD was carefully inserted and checked for any excessive soft-tissue contact and compression in order to guarantee uneventful healing. Besides assuring function, phonetics, and esthetics, the objective was to establish slight soft-tissue contact, especially at the interproximal aspects, to provide minimal support to the papillary tissue, preventing excessive collapse towards the center of the extraction site (Fig 10).

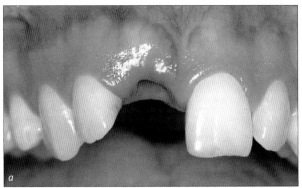 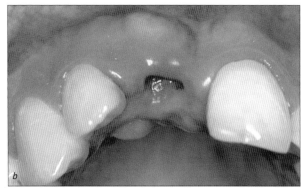

Figs 11a, b   Vestibular (a) and occlusal (b) views of the extraction site six weeks after the right central maxillary incisor had been removed. Only minimal soft-tissue loss in an orofacial and a coronoapical direction could be observed, and the scalloped course of the gingival was maintained. A marked concavity still existed in the center of the former extraction site.

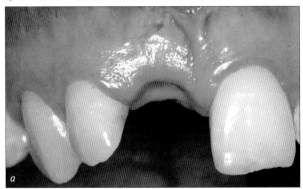 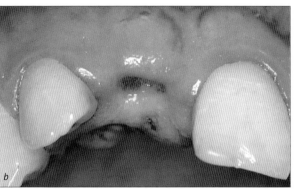

Figs 12a, b   Eight weeks after the extraction of tooth 11, the soft-tissue situation at the site of implantation was considered adequate according to the preferred early placement/early loading protocol.

Six weeks after the extraction, the soft tissue of the future implant site had uneventfully healed and the respective wound surface was completely epithelialized (Figs 11a, b). As expected, only minimal loss of soft-tissue height at the interproximal aspects and of soft-tissue width in an orofacial direction was observed. The harmonious course of the gingiva could largely be maintained.

However, as a distinct concavity at the center of the former extraction site was still present, it was decided to wait for more tissue fill-in and to postpone the planned insertion of the implant for an additional two weeks.

This additional healing time contributed to a more favorable soft-tissue situation from a surgical point of view, eight weeks after the extraction (Figs 12a, b).

At this stage, a periapical radiograph was taken to examine the osseous status at the future implantation site (Fig 13). This two-dimensional diagnostic document confirmed that the vertical bone level at the interproximal aspects of the two neighboring teeth was maintained at a

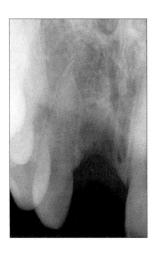

Fig 13   Eight-week post-extraction apical radiograph documenting favorable bone height at the interproximal aspects of the adjacent teeth.

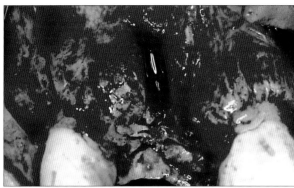

Fig 14   After elevation of a mucoperiosteal flap with mesial and distal relieving incisions, the absence of the buccal bone plate at the center of the prospective implantation site became apparent.

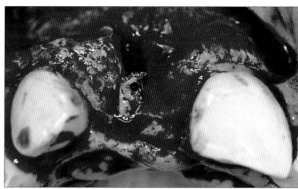

Fig 15   Occlusal view, confirming that only moderate horizontal bone loss had occurred since the extraction.

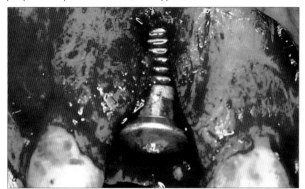

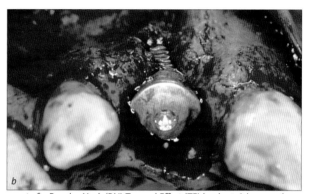

Figs 16a, b   Labial (a) and occlusal (b) views of site 11 immediately after placement of a Regular Neck (RN) Tapered Effect (TE) implant. Adequate three-dimensional implant position, completely within the alveolar housing and fully compatible with a simultaneous localized GBR procedure.

height similar to that before the tooth was removed. As this height corresponded to a physiological distance from the CEJ of the adjacent teeth and as this parameter had been proven to represent a key factor for soft-tissue support around implants, the esthetic prognosis was excellent.

Based on the clinical and radiographic examinations that had confirmed that the optimal situation for early implant placement had been reached, the decision was made to proceed to the surgical phase of the treatment. A slightly palatal crestal incision was chosen and a mucoperiosteal flap with two relieving incisions was elevated. As expected, part of the buccal bone plate was missing, but without affecting the width of the orofacial crest at adjacent teeth further apically (Fig 14).

The occlusal view of the site confirmed, as anticipated, the compatibility of the local crestal-bone anatomy with the placement of an implant in combination with a simultaneous guided bone regeneration (GBR) procedure (Fig 15). More specifically, a localized bone defect at the vestibular aspect of the prospective implant site was ob-

served. This favorable two-wall defect anatomy is fully compatible with the insertion of an implant, as it permits the achievement of (1) primary implant stability; (2) an implant position entirely inside of the alveolar crest confinement; and (3) either a three-wall or a two-wall defect that can be corrected predictably with a simultaneous GBR procedure.

As documented by Figures 16a and b, an adequate three-dimensional implant position, resulting in a two-wall bony defect at the buccal aspect, was achieved. The entire circumference of the implant body and the implant shoulder were located within the alveolar bone crest (Buser and coworkers, 2004).

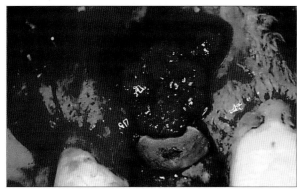

Fig 17   The persisting localized dehiscence-type defect on the labial aspect of the freshly inserted implant was covered with small bone chips harvested next to the implant site.

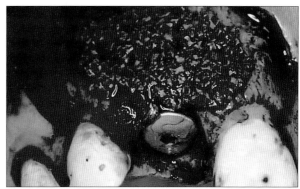

Fig 18   With the application of a substantial layer of bone fillers on the localization of the dehiscence defect, which gradually extended to the periphery, a distinct convexity at site 11 was achieved. This procedure, which included a slight "overbuild" of the vestibular contour of the alveolar bone crest, was intended to provide the required support and long-term stability for the overlaying soft tissue.

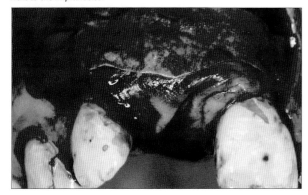

Fig 19   A bioabsorbable barrier membrane was applied in two layers to create the preconditions for a successful GBR-procedure. No additional membrane-fixation measures were necessary.

Once the appropriate three-dimensional implant position had been reached and its primary stability confirmed, the localized GBR procedure was undertaken. It consisted first of the harvesting of autogenous bone grafts ("chips") in the close vicinity of the implant site and then of an adaptation to the exposed buccal implant surface to fill in the small dehiscence-type defect (Fig 17).

In order to guarantee an adequate thickness of the buccal bone wall, a substantial layer of bone fillers, soaked in blood, was applied (Fig 18). These bone fillers with a lowsubstitution rate will provide the necessary support and stability for the overlaying soft tissue. As the bone fillers would be resorbed only slowly or not at all, the convex vestibular alveolar-ridge profile achieved strongly resembled that normally observed buccally of natural roots, would be maintainable long term.

As well documented in the literature, a bioabsorbable barrier membrane was applied to avoid a second open-flap procedure to remove the membrane. A so-called "double-layer" technique was used to improve membrane stability. Once soaked with blood, the membranes could easily be adapted to the alveolar-bone crest and did not require any additional fixation (Fig 19). In the esthetic zone, complete soft-tissue coverage of the implant site is most often preferred, in combination with a submerged approach aimed at complete primary wound closure.

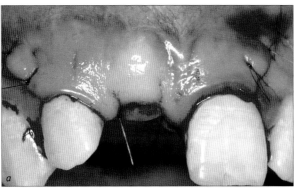 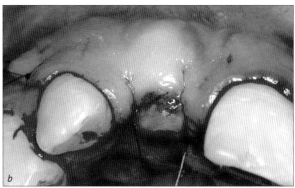

Figs 20a, b   Primary wound closure was achieved with incision of the periosteum at the basal level of the flap, compensating for the significant "over-build" of the labial aspect at the implant site.

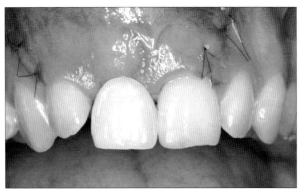 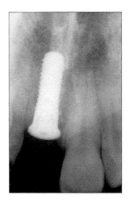

Fig 21   Periapical radiograph, illustrating a satisfactory position of the implant with respect to the different landmarks (CEJ, neighboring roots) provided by the adjacent natural dentition.

Fig 22   The provisional RPD was shortened at site 11 to minimize the risk of interference with the healing process.

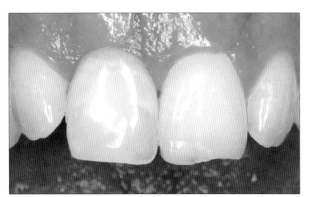

Fig 23   As soon as the process of soft-tissue healing permitted, the temporary RPD was carefully relined to establish optimal tissue contact and to improve the esthetic appearance of the anterior maxilla.

In order to permit optimal, tension-free flap adaptation in view of a complete primary wound closure (Figs 20a, b), the periosteum was split at the basis of the flap.

At the end of the surgical procedure, an apical radiograph was taken to serve as a baseline reference and to document/verify the adequate relationship between the neighboring roots and the intrabony part of the inserted implant (Fig 21).

The GBR procedure required a significant cervical reduction of the provisional RPD to avoid any excessive tissue compression in the region of the freshly inserted implant (Fig 22).

After ten days of uneventful soft-tissue healing, the temporary restoration was relined for the patient's subjective comfort and to improve the esthetic appearance in the region of the anterior maxilla (Fig 23).

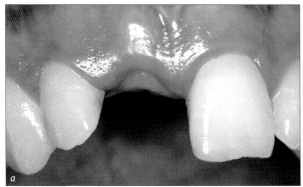
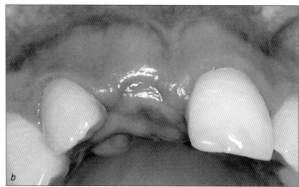

Figs 24a, b   Vestibular (a) and occlusal (b) of the implant site after a ten-week period of uneventful healing, documenting that the first phase of post surgical soft-tissue maturation was completed. Only minimal vertical tissue loss had occurred compared with the pre-surgical situation.

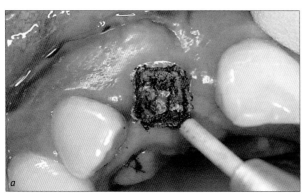
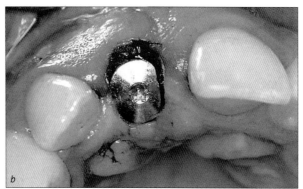

Figs 26a, b   A CO_2 laser technique was applied to create access to the underlying implant shoulder (a). The original short healing cap was subsequently replaced by a longer one to maintain the newly established restorative access (b).

In accordance with an early loading protocol and taking into account the individual extent of GBR performed, the prosthodontic procedure could be initiated in this patient ten weeks after implant placement. At that time, the phase of primary soft-tissue healing was considered completed (Figs 24a, b).

A periapical radiograph was taken to confirm a stable peri-implant bone situation (Fig 25). In particular, the interproximal height of the bone surrounding the adjacent natural teeth had been maintained at a level comparable to that before implant placement.

The first step of the restorative phase consisted of establishing access from the soft-tissue surface to the underlying implant shoulder. In this patient, a CO_2 laser technique (Fig 26a) was used and the short titanium healing cap replaced with a longer one (Fig 26b) in order to maintain the freshly created restorative access.

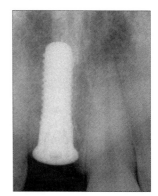

Fig 25   Intraoral radiograph, documenting the anticipated stable peri-implant bone.

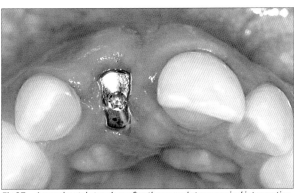

Fig 27   Approximately ten days after the second-stage surgical intervention, the soft tissue allowed proceeding to the next prosthodontic step.

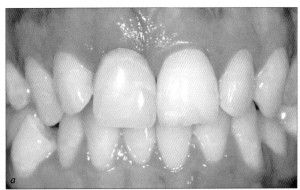

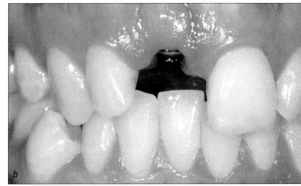

Figs 28a, b   Comparison of the labial views with (a) and without (b) the provisional RPD, indicating that sufficient soft-tissue height was present at site 11 to create a symmetrical soft-tissue contour at the position of the two central maxillary incisors.

Ten days later, the peri-implant soft tissue (Fig 27) was considered compatible with impression-taking or the fabrication of a chairside implant-supported provisional restoration.

A direct comparison between the labial view with (Fig 28a) and without (Fig 28b) the provisional RPD in place gave rise to the expectation that the slight excess in soft-tissue height at site 11 would be sufficient to ultimately create a restoration emergence profile similar to that of the contralateral tooth (21).

It was decided to proceed to the fabrication of a direct fixed implant-supported provisional in an attempt to establish optimal peri-implant soft-tissue contours prior to the implant impression. For the fabrication of the planned chairside provisional, a newly developed restorative component, the Regular Neck (RN) synOcta temporary mesoabutment, was used (Fig 29). It is possible to add acrylic resin directly to this substructure, fabricating a one-piece screw-retained implant provisional. The same component can also be used as a mesostructure, serving as a base for a cemented provisional restoration. This component could also be utilized — after substantial occlusal reduction — as a screw-retained tissue conditioner/healing abutment. Under these circumstances, a patient would continue to wear his or her provisional RPD.

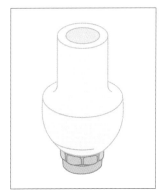

Fig 29   The RN synOcta temporary meso-abutment was used for chairside fabrication of an occlusally screw-retained temporary implant-supported crown. As the marginal area is prefabricated, the clinician only needed to adapt the cervical emergence profile (subtractively or additively) to the requirements of the clinical situation.

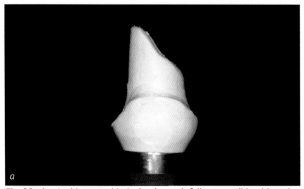
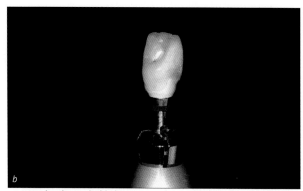

Figs 30a, b   In this case, with the implant axis fully compatible with occlusal screw retention, it was decided to connect the provisional crown directly to the implant. As the cervical part of the component is prefabricated and has an excellent marginal fit by definition, a significant number of the fabrication steps can be performed extraorally.

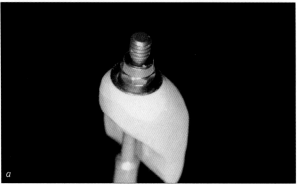
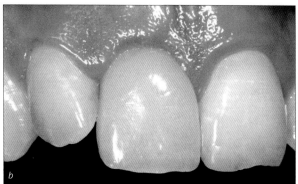

Figs 31a, b   After finishing and polishing, the temporary crown (a) produced at chairside was ready for insertion (b).

The component described could subsequently be attached to a corresponding implant analog, facilitating the finishing procedures that were performed extraorally (Fig 30a). A special holder (Fig 30b) is available for the fixation of the analog.

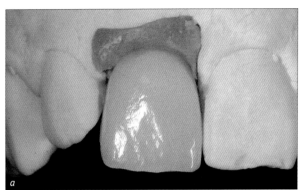

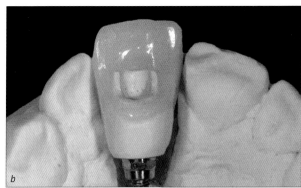

Figs 32a, b   For demonstration purposes, a screw-retained provisional crown was fabricated in the dental laboratory, using the previously described RN syn-Octa temporary mesoabutment as its base.

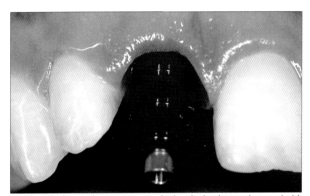

Fig 33   The impression cap was attached to the implant and secured with the matching occlusal screw. The peri-implant soft-tissue contours were satisfactory

The RN synOcta temporary mesoabutment can also be used as a base for a screw-retained provisional crown fabricated on a working cast in the dental laboratory (Figs 32a, b).

Two months after the insertion of the fixed temporary implant restoration, the peri-implant soft-tissue contours were judged to be adequate, so that the clinical situation was ripe for taking the final impression. As the implant shoulder was located distinctly submucosally, particularly at the mesial and distal aspects, an approach involving a screw-retained impression cap and an open tray was preferred (Fig 33).

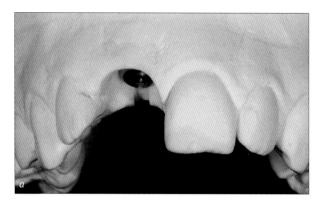

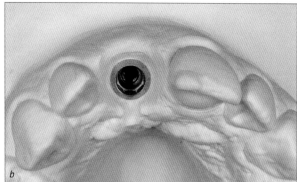

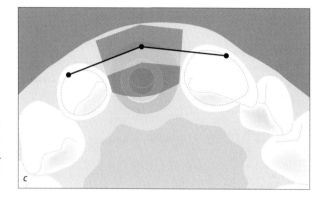

Figs 34a-c   Vestibular (a) and occlusal (b) views of the master cast, showing a satisfactory three-dimensional implant position and peri-implant soft-tissue contours optimized on the working cast by the laboratory technician. An access slot was created at the palatal aspect for better visual control of the margin and for ease of manipulation. The implant is ideally placed within the orofacial and mesiodistal comfort zones (c).

A stone working model was produced to fabricate an occlusally screw-retained permanent implant-supported crown (Figs 34a, b).

The master cast was reproduced in a special dental stone that provided the strong optical contrast necessary for the scanning process essential to Straumann CARES, the Computer Aided REstoration Service (Fig 35).

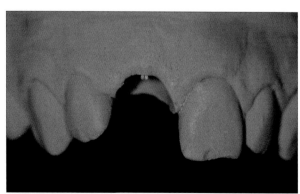

Fig 35   Labial view of the working cast with the increased optical contrast required for the CARES system during the scanning process.

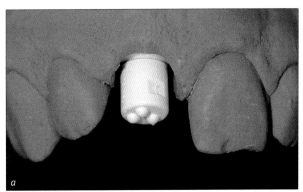 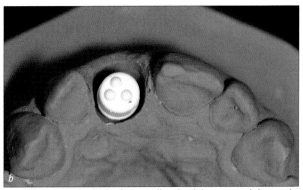

Figs 36a, b   Labial and occlusal close-up views of implant site 11 after attachment of the scanbody with its three small occlusal domes, permitting precise three-dimensional scanning of the implant shoulder position.

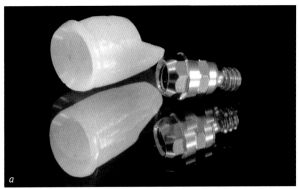 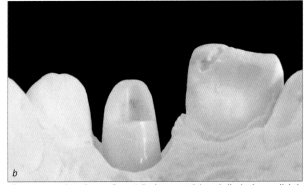

Figs 37a, b   The computer-generated zirconium-dioxide custom abutment, to be connected to the synOcta 1.5 abutment (a) and displaying a slightly "whitish" appearance (b), required some preliminary modification to create optimal conditions for esthetic ceramic veneering.

The so-called scanbody, a prefabricated system component with three well-defined domes at its occlusal aspect, was attached to the implant analog at site 11 by simple finger pressure (Figs 36a, b). The master cast was thus ready to be inserted into the InEos scanner (Sirona) for automatic digitizing of the precise three-dimensional implant shoulder position.

After the scanning process, the three-dimensional outline of an optimal all-ceramic (ZrO_2) CARES custom abutment was designed on the computer screen and milled by the respective computer-assisted manufacturing (CAM) unit. This ceramic custom abutment (Fig 37a) connected to a synOcta 1.5 abutment and allowed for direct veneering with adapted feldspathic ceramics (Fig 37b).

Although the zirconium-dioxide custom abutment featured a certain degree of translucency, its slightly "whitish" appearance (Fig 38a) made a minor preliminary color modification necessary, creating a more dentine-like appearance (Fig 38b) and facilitating the subsequent esthetic veneering (Andersson and coworkers, 2001).

Despite the addition of this dentine-like ceramic layer, a significant degree of translucency could be maintained, which was verified by light transmission (Fig 39).

In the dental laboratory, the ceramist had the demanding task of duplicating as closely as possible the optical properties of the natural left maxillary central incisor (contralateral tooth) by applying a complex layering technique and anticipating the significant volume contraction associated with the subsequent sintering process (Figs 40a, b).

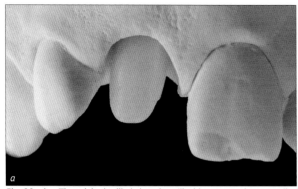 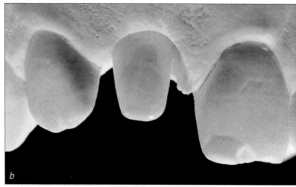

Figs 38a, b   The original milled zirconium-dioxide custom abutment displayed a slightly "whitish" appearance (a). Therefore, a first layer of a more dentine-like ceramic material was applied (b) to create an appropriate base for the subsequent layers of ceramic veneering.

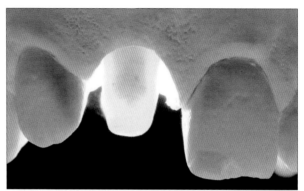

Fig 39   After adding a thin layer of dentine-like ceramic, the remaining translucency of the ZrO$_2$ custom abutment was verified under light-transmission conditions.

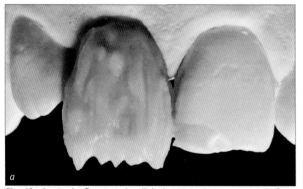 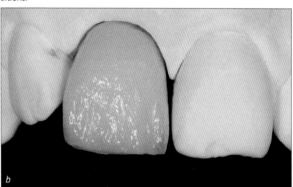

Figs 40a, b   In the first step, the clinical crown volume, composed of a complex sequence of layers of different opacities and shades, imitating the basic components—dentine, enamel, and incisal translucency—of a natural maxillary incisor, was established (a). After the first ceramic sintering, a significant volume contraction was observed, requiring at least one additional corrective step. The basic optical properties, however, were already clearly discernible.

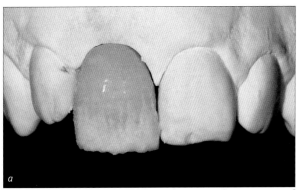 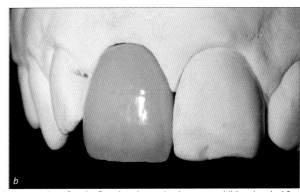

Figs 41a, b   Precise addition of more translucent ceramic to compensate for the contraction after the first sintering and to integrate additional optical features from the contralateral natural tooth (a). After the second sintering process, some minor finishing with rotary instruments was performed before the subsequent clinical try-in (b).

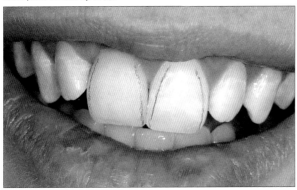

Fig 42   The first clinical try-in of the all-ceramic implant-supported crown 11 revealed an acceptable integration into its natural surroundings and confirmed that the basic features of tooth and tooth volume and the localization of the mesial and distal transition line angles had closely duplicated those of contralateral natural tooth.

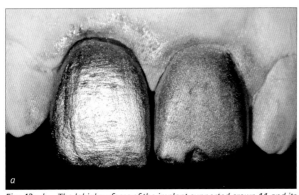 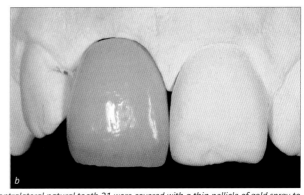

Figs 43a, b   The labial surfaces of the implant-supported crown 11 and its contralateral natural tooth 21 were covered with a thin pellicle of gold spray to better highlight the basic features of tooth form and surface texture (a). This facilitated the last finishing steps, mainly carried out by rotary instruments (b).

Minute layers of more translucent ceramic material were added where necessary to compensate for the contraction that had occurred after the first sintering process (Fig 41a). After this second sintering process, followed by some final adjustments with rotary instruments, the implant-supported crown was ready for the clinical try-in (Fig 41b).

A clinical try-in of the ceramic implant-supported crown in its "biscuit stage" was needed to identify, by comparing the natural tooth and the ceramic crown, the optical and esthetic key parameters, such as interproximal ridges, mesial and distal transition line angles, and surface characteristics (Fig 42).

In the dental laboratory, the final modifications, focusing primarily on the surface texture characteristics as seen in the contralateral natural tooth, were carried out (Figs 43a, b)

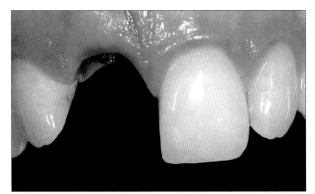

Fig 44   Labial view of the anterior maxilla after replacing the existing mesioincisal composite restoration.

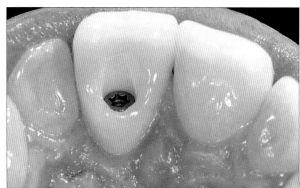

Fig 46   Palatal view of the newly inserted all ceramic implant-supported crown, showing that despite the considerable height and volume of this restoration type, a satisfactory contour was achieved compared to the adjacent dentition.

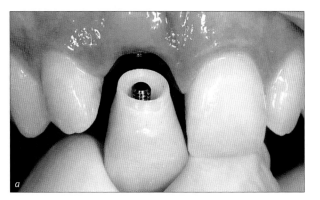

a

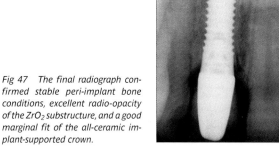

Fig 47   The final radiograph confirmed stable peri-implant bone conditions, excellent radio-opacity of the ZrO_2 substructure, and a good marginal fit of the all-ceramic implant-supported crown.

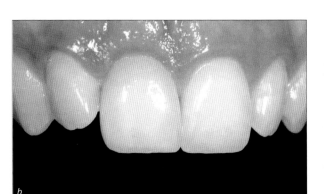

b

Figs 45a, b   The all-ceramic implant-supported crown 11 was inserted (a) and its esthetic integration verified (b).

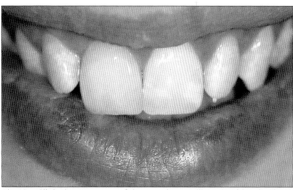

Fig 48   Clinical appearance of the anterior maxillary dentition (patient's unforced smile).

At this stage, the existing composite restoration at the mesioincisal angle of tooth 21 was replaced (Fig 44). The final all-ceramic crown was inserted and its occlusal screw tightened to 15 Ncm (Fig 45), and the screw-access channel was closed with composite resin.

The radiographic control confirmed stable bony peri-implant conditions, excellent radio-opacity of the zirconium-dioxide custom abutment, and adequate marginal adaptation of the all-ceramic implant-supported crown (Fig 47).

The patient's unforced smile at the end of treatment documented that the implant-supported crown blended in nicely with the surrounding natural dentition, matching quite satisfactorily the adjacent natural teeth in shape, texture, and color. Furthermore, the line of the marginal gingiva and the line of the incisal edges in relation to the border of the lower lip were harmonious (Fig 48).

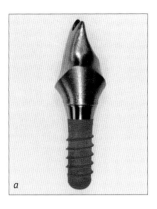

Figs 49a, b   For direct comparison, an additional CARES titanium custom abutment (a) was produced for this same implant, serving as a base for a cemented Auro-Galvano ceramo-metal crown (b).

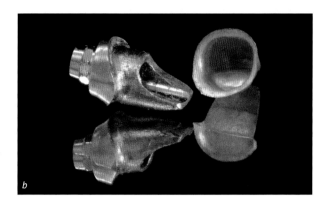

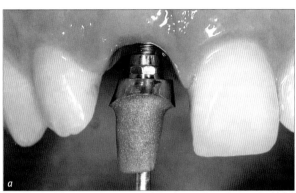

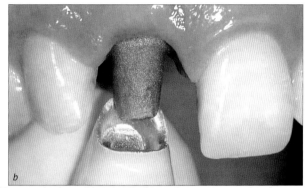

Figs 50a, b   The computer-generated titanium custom abutment, which had been previously sandblasted at the future abutment-to-crown interface, was connected directly to implant 11 and subsequently tightened to 35 Ncm (a). The cemented ceramo-metal crown was then tried in (b).

For demonstration and direct comparison purposes, a second crown was produced for implant 11 based on a CARES titanium custom abutment directly connected to the underlying implant (Figs 49 – 52).

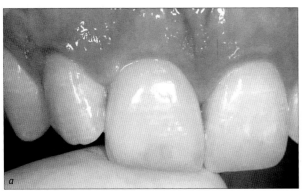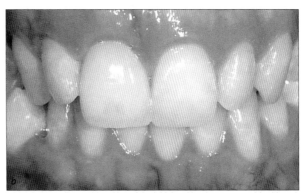

Fig 51a,b   The implant-supported crown was held in place with light finger pressure, which led to a discrete blanching of the labial peri-implant mucosa (a). Although still largely acceptable from an esthetic point of view, this second ceramo-metal crown — in contrast to the all-ceramic crown presented previously — showed a slight "grayish" shadow along the labial soft-tissue margin (b). This optical phenomenon was probably due to a decrease in light transmission caused by the metal framework.

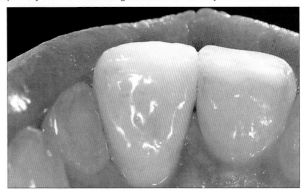

Fig 52   The palatal view, however, demonstrated the more favorable cervical configuration of this type of implant-supported crown, which does not require a screw-access channel.

Acknowledgments

Surgical Procedures
Dr. Daniel Buser – Professor, University of Bern, Switzerland, Department of Oral Surgery and Stomatology

Laboratory Procedures
Master Dental Technician Dominique Vinci, University of Geneva, Switzerland

4.6   Replacement of an Upper Right Central Incisor with a Regular Neck Implant, Restored with an All-Ceramic Crown, Cemented

R. Jung

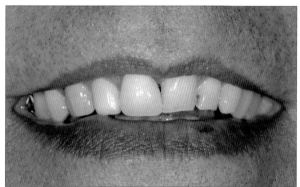

Fig 1   At medium smile, the patient displayed at least three-quarters of his incisors. The incisal edges were unharmonious.

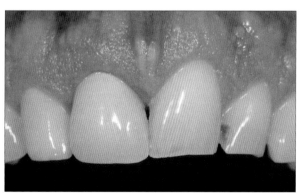

Fig 2   Buccal view of the incisors revealing a thick-tissue biotype with soft-tissue excess to the buccal gingival margin of tooth 11.

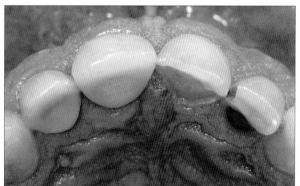

Fig 3   Occlusal view of the incisors. Favorable buccal contour.

The 54-year-old male patient, a non-smoker, had ceramo-metal crowns on teeth 11 and 12 that no longer met his esthetic needs (Fig 1). The patient was free of pain. His medical history was without significant findings, and the patient was in good general health.

The patient's wish was to improve the esthetics of his anterior teeth.

At full smile, the patient presented a medium to high lip line, displaying the full crowns and the marginal gingiva (Fig 1).

The harmony of the gingival margin was disrupted by the now rejected ceramo-metal crowns on teeth 11 and 12. The crowns differed from the respective contralateral teeth in shape, texture, and color (Fig 2).

The patient's gingival biotype was thick, with a broad band of attached keratinized gingiva and a moderate (medium) scallop height.

The soft tissues were free of recessions (Fig 2). The patient's soft-tissue situation was favorable due to the slight soft-tissue excess at the buccal gingival margin of tooth 11 compared to that of tooth 21.

The patient's crown shape was mostly triangular. The more the crown shape tends towards the triangular, the higher the esthetic risk. In this patient, however, the esthetic risk was reduced thanks to the contact area that was present at the mesial aspect of tooth 21. Furthermore, the incisal edges of the contralateral teeth differed in height. Teeth 11 and 12 appeared to be longer than the respective contralateral teeth. The option to shorten the incisal portion of a tooth reduces the esthetic risk of obtaining a long clinical crown after implant reconstruction.

The incisal view shows a harmoniously contoured arch without any horizontal deficiencies (Fig 3).

A loose crown on tooth 11 was detected at the clinical examination. Further, the pre-treatment periapical radiograph revealed a root-canal filling and secondary caries at tooth 11, which was also fractured in the coronal part of its root (Fig 4).

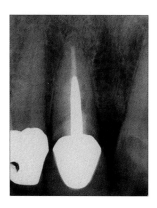

Fig 4   Periapical radiograph showing a root-canal filled tooth with a post and a gap between the crown and the root. The periapical area seemed to have no pathology, and the interproximal bone level of the adjacent teeth seemed to be intact.

Radiologically, the interproximal bone-crest levels of the adjacent teeth seemed to be sufficiently well maintained to allow for a distance of about 5 mm between them and the contact points of the future crowns (Fig 5).

If the distance between the interproximal bone crest and the contact point exceeds 5 mm, the papilla may not fill the interdental space, and a "black triangle" is likely to result (Tarnow and coworkers, 1992; Choquet and coworkers, 2001).

Periodontal probing revealed a probing depth of 6 mm at the buccal aspect of tooth 11. This might be explained by the superficial fracture of the buccal root. Mesially, the probing depth exceeded 5 mm; more tissue could have been lost during therapy, a fact that needed to be taken into account. The patient needed to be informed about this clinical finding and its potential influence on the esthetic treatment outcome, as it created an esthetic risk.

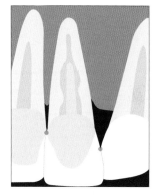

Fig 5   Interproximal bone-crest levels of the adjacent teeth allowing the "5-mm rule" to be observed.

The gingival margin of contralateral tooth 21 was located about 1.5 mm further apically than that of tooth 11. This "soft-tissue excess" around tooth 11 in combination with the medium-scalloped, thick-tissue biotype were important prerequisites for immediate implant placement and transmucosal healing.

After immediate implant placement, unpredictable remodeling processes at the hard-tissue and soft-tissue level had to be expected (Botticelli and coworkers, 2004). Favorable conditions as in this patient (Fig 6) will tolerate a certain amount of soft-tissue recession without compromising the esthetic treatment outcome.

The above clinical and radiological findings are the basis for the patient's esthetic risk profile (Table 1):

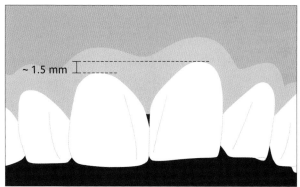

~ 1.5 mm

Fig 6   Soft-tissue excess at the future implant site minimizing the risk of a compromised esthetic treatment outcome with regard to the height of the future peri-implant mucosa.

Table 1 The patient's individual esthetic risk profile.

Esthetic Risk Factors	Low	Medium	High
Medical status	Healthy, cooperative patient with intact immune system		
Smoking habit	Non-smoker		
Patient's esthetic expectations		Medium	
Lip line		Medium	
Gingival biotype	thick	Medium scalloped,	
Shape of tooth crowns			Triangular
Infection at implant site	None		
Bone level at adjacent teeth		5.5 to 6.5 mm to contact point	
Restorative status of neighboring teeth			Restored
Width of edentulous span	1 tooth (≥ 7 mm)		
Soft-tissue anatomy	Intact soft tissue		
Bone anatomy of alveolar crest	Alveolar crest without bone deficiency		

The esthetic risk-profile analysis shows a medium esthetic risk for this patient.

Based on the above analysis, it was decided to extract tooth 11 in a minimally invasive mode and to perform immediate implant placement (type 1) with transmucosal implant healing, using a Standard Plus implant with an endosseous diameter of 4.1 mm and a Regular Neck prosthetic platform of 4.8 mm in diameter and 12 mm in length. Figure 7 shows the pre-implantation treatment planning on the orthopantomograph (OPT).

For immediate implant placement, it was important to have at least about 3 mm of residual bone height apically of the extraction socket to ensure sufficient primary stability (Fig 7).

Because the root of the extracted tooth 11 was tilted distally, the implant bed had to be carefully prepared regarding the mesiodistal aspect of the extraction socket to ensure a correct three-dimensional position of the implant (Figs 10, 11).

In order to ensure optimal access to the implant site and the expected buccal bone deficiency and to keep bone denudation and soft-tissue trauma as minimal as possible, a flap design with one vertical releasing incision at the distal aspect of adjacent tooth 12 was chosen (Fig 8)

A TE (Tapered Effect) implant would have been a sound choice as well, but at the time of implantation, the TE implant was not yet commercially available.

Immediately after tooth extraction, the implant was placed according to the desired prosthetic treatment outcome, i.e. the future line of the marginal mucosa (top-down approach) (Figs 9, 10).

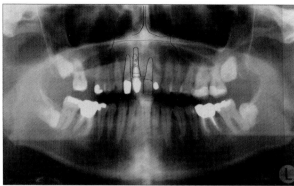

Fig 7   Visualization of preoperative treatment planning by drawing the adjacent roots, the anatomical structures, and the planned implant on a transparent foil on top of the OPT.

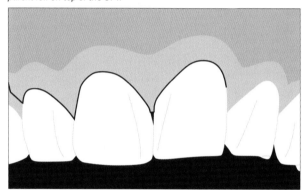

Fig 8   One vertical releasing incision instead of two to reduce trauma and the area of bone denudation.

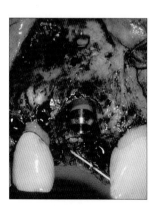

Fig 9   The implant after placement in a correct coronoapical position.

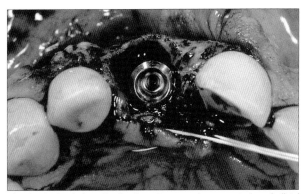

Fig 10   Occlusal view after implant placement in a corrected mesiodistal dimension (note the discrepancy between root form and position and the implant form and position).

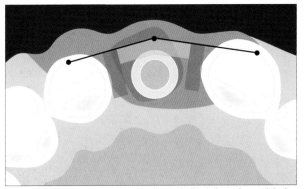

Fig 11   The implant was centered in the mesiodistal dimension and the implant shoulder was located in the orofacial comfort zone.

When it comes to placing an immediate implant in an extraction socket, special care needs to be taken to prepare the implant bed in the ideal three-dimensional position. It may be helpful to plan and drill as if the extraction-socket defect were not present. In this case, this led to an implant position in the mesiopalatal aspect of the extraction socket (Figs 10, 11).

The horizontal bone deficiency, including the apical fenestration defect, was covered with a deproteinized bone allograft (Fig 12), and the site was subsequently covered with a resorbable collagen membrane stabilized with two resorbable polylactide pins (Fig 13).

The fixation of the membrane served to maintain the desired shape and prevented the membrane and allograft material from dislocating.

After a periosteal releasing incision, the flap was carefully mobilized, repositioned free of tension, and sutured with non-resorbable suture material, allowing the implant to heal in a semi-submerged mode (Fig 14). The use of a labially beveled healing cap allowed the placement of the buccal flap slightly further coronally to provide for soft-tissue excess at the prospective implant site.

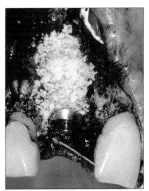

Fig 12   Buccal view after augmentation with a membrane-supporting material. The site was slightly overcontoured to ensure an adequate buccal root prominence after treatment.

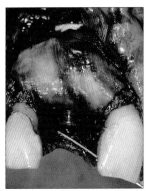

Fig 13   Buccal view after positioning and tacking the collagen membrane.

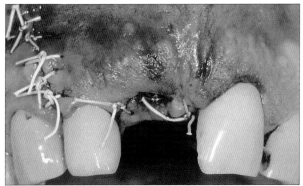

Fig 14   Buccal view after repositioning the flap to allow for a semi-submerged healing mode.

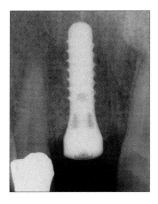

Fig 15   The radiograph after twelve weeks of healing showing successful implant integration.

Four weeks after implant placement, the clinical situation was inconspicuous (Figs 16, 17). Some soft-tissue excess was still present at the buccal aspect of the labially beveled healing cap (Figs 16, 17), which facilitated subsequent soft-tissue conditioning.

Twelve weeks after implant placement, the healing cap was removed for impression-taking.

The small cylindrical area of access to the implant would not yet allow the insertion of a crown with its final emergence profile (Fig 18).

Either a larger healing cap or a temporary crown may be used for soft-tissue conditioning. For diagnostic reasons, a temporary crown has multiple advantages in the esthetic area, such as soft-tissue conditioning, evaluation of crown length and profile, phonetic checks, and the patient's overall acceptance of and coping with the implant reconstruction.

Figs 19 and 20 show the situation with the impression cap carefully screwed into place (hand-tight).

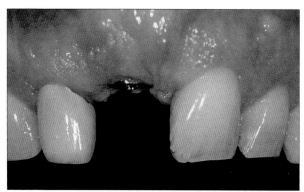
Fig 16   Buccal view of implant site 11 still showing some soft-tissue excess compared to the contralateral tooth.

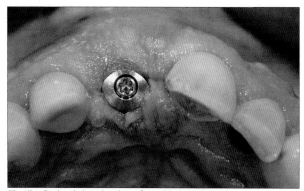
Fig 17   Occlusal view showing a favorable buccal contour.

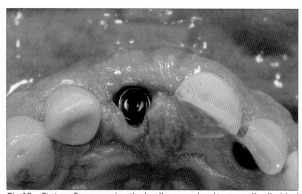
Fig 18   Status after removing the healing cap, showing a small cylindrical area of access to the implant.

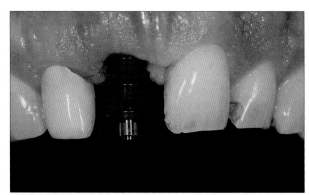
Fig 20   Buccal view of the impression cap.

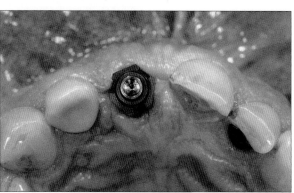
Fig 19   Occlusal view of the impression cap.

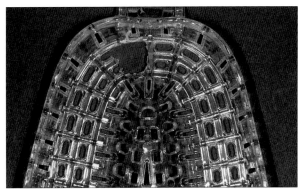

Fig 21   Customized tray with the access hole at site 11.

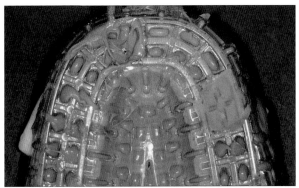

Fig 22   Impression tray with polyether impression material.

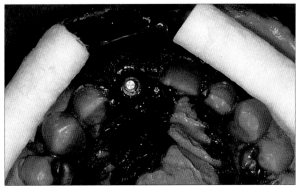

Fig 23   Impression ready for transfer to the dental lab.

In order to facilitate the use of a screw-retained impression cap, a customized tray was modified at site 11 so it allowed for screw access (Fig 21).

After complete setting of the impression material, the screw of the impression cap was loosened through the custom-made impression tray's access hole for removal of the impression (Fig 22).

Based upon that impression (Fig 23), a master model was fabricated in the dental lab on which a custom temporary crown was to be fabricated.

To avoid multiple cementation of the temporary crown for soft-tissue conditioning, a screw-retained crown was produced, using a titanium post for temporary restorations (Fig 24).

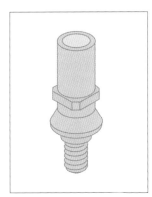

Fig 24   synOcta post for temporary restorations, titanium.

After defining the final form and dimension of the crown in wax, a silicone key was made. The post was tightened on the implant analog and trimmed to the desired height. The silicone key served to determine the ideal occlusal height (Fig 25).

After sandblasting, silanization, and sealing the screw channel, an opaque was applied, and the screw-retained temporary crown was layered with a self-curing resin material (polymethyl methacrylate, PMMA) and characterized with light-curing composite.

Using a self-curing PMMA for the provisional crown, the dentine core of the crown was condensed and pressure-cured, resulting in the crown's dentine "core." This dentine core was then characterized using light-curing composite shades. PMMA for the incisal crown portion was added, giving the crown its final tooth shape. It is important that all the composite colors applied to the dentine core be covered with PMMA for the incisal crown portion.

Special attention was paid in order to create an ideal emergence profile and crown shape in harmony with that of the contralateral tooth. A silicone gingiva mask facilitated the creation of the emergence profile (Figs 26, 27).

Fig 28 shows the clinical situation immediately after insertion of the provisional crown, thirteen weeks after implantation. The transocclusally screw-retained provisional crown was placed in the implant's internal octagon and tightened by hand.

In order not to traumatize the tissue, a chairside reduction of the cervical crown dimension is often needed to allow insertion of the temporary crown.

Note the blanching of the mucosa due to the pressure applied by the crown (Fig 28).

This pressure initiates the mucosa-conditioning phase.

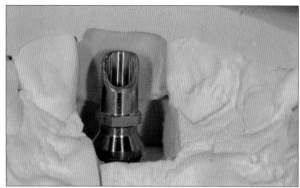

Fig 25   synOcta titanium post, customized for the clinical situation according to the diagnostic waxup.

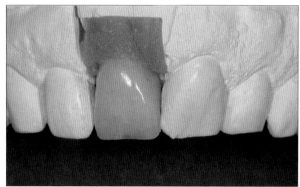

Fig 26   Buccal view of the final provisional crown.

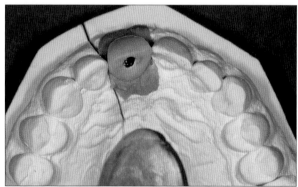

Fig 27   Occlusal view of the final provisional crown.

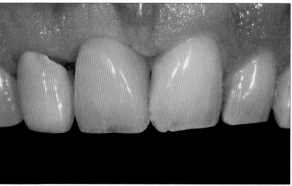

Fig 28   The provisional crown was inserted with slight pressure on the peri-implant mucosa.

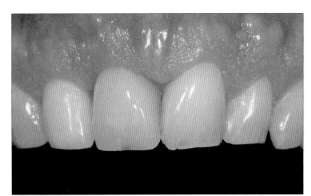

Fig 29   Buccal view of the temporary crown, three weeks after insertion.

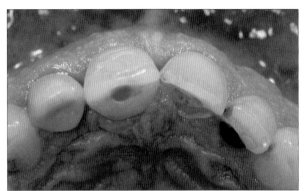

Fig 30   Occlusal view of the temporary crown, three weeks after insertion.

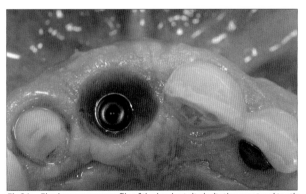

Fig 31   Final emergence profile of the implant site imitating a natural tooth profile.

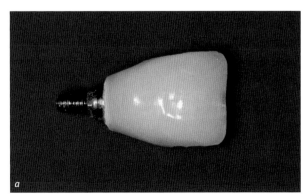

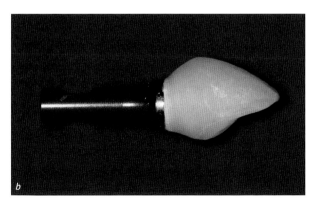

Figs 32a, b   The temporary crown (a) screwed onto an implant analog (b).

Three weeks later, the mucosa was healthy and stable (Figs 29, 30). It had nicely adapted to the emergence profile of the implant-supported temporary crown. Meanwhile, the ceramo-metal crown on tooth 12 was replaced by an acrylic temporary crown. Note the improved papilla contours to the distal of tooth 11 as well as between teeth 11 and 21.

During the soft-tissue conditioning phase, the emergence profile of the temporary crown was adapted twice, three and six weeks after its first attachment to the implant. Depending on the diameter of the tooth and the resistance of the mucosa, one to three conditioning steps should be planned for.

The maturation of the soft tissue around an implant crown takes place within the first three to six months after insertion of the reconstruction (Grunder, 2000). Hence, a minimum time of three months after insertion of the temporary crown should be allowed for soft-tissue maturation and stabilization.

Four months after first insertion, the desired final emergence profile was achieved (Fig 31), and the mucosa was shaped according to the contours of the final provisional (Fig 32).

To capture and transfer the emergence profile as precisely as possible by means of a second impression intended for the fabrication of the master model for the final crown, the final temporary crown was screwed onto an implant analog (Hinds 1997) (Fig 32).

The implant analog and the temporary crown were inserted into putty silicone material to capture the shape of the crown's cervical portion (Fig 33).

After the silicone had set, the crown was removed by loosening the occlusal screw so that a precise copy of its cervical shape was captured within the silicone (Fig 34).

A screw-retained impression cap was seated on the analog and tightened. The gap between the silicone and the impression cap was filled with a flowable light-curing composite (Fig 35).

The result was an individualized impression cap that exactly mimicked the temporary crown's cervical portion (Fig 36).

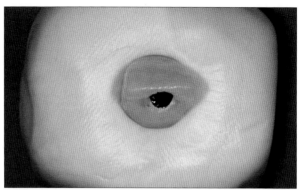

Fig 33   Temporary crown inserted into putty silicone material up to about one-half of the crown.

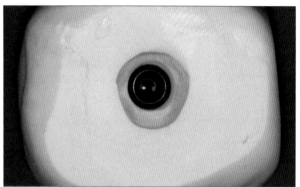

Fig 34   Cervical shape of the temporary crown as captured within the silicone.

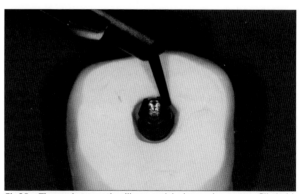

Fig 35   The gap between the silicone and the impression cap was filled with a flowable light curing composite.

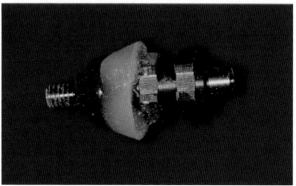

Fig 36   Individualized impression cap mimicking the final emergence profile.

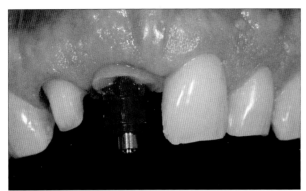

Fig 37   Individualized impression cap ideally supporting the mucosa.

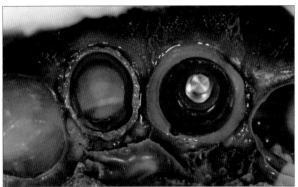

Fig 38   Final impression. Favorable situation at tooth 12 and implant site 11.

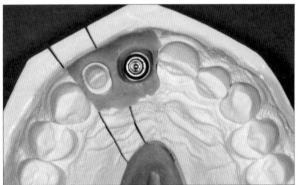

Fig 39   Final master cast for the tooth-supported crown 12 and the implant-supported crown 11.

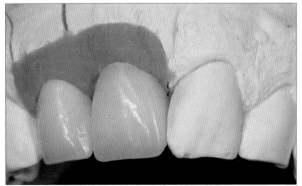

Fig 40   Diagnostic waxup crowns for teeth 12 and 11.

This individualized impression cap not only prevented the conditioned peri-implant mucosa from collapsing when the temporary was removed, but it also provided ideal support for the mucosa during impression-taking (Fig 37) and captured the ideal emergence profile within the impression (Fig 38).

The result was a new, definitive master model that precisely captured the shape of the peri-implant mucosa, communicating the diagnostic findings and past clinical procedure to the dental technician (Fig 39).

To determine the ideal shape and dimensions of the final crowns, a waxup was produced (Fig 40).

2.1.3   Statements C: Prosthodontic and Restorative Procedures

Statement C.1
Standards for an Esthetic Fixed Implant Restoration
An esthetic implant prosthesis was defined as one that is in harmony with the peri-oral facial structures of the patient. The esthetic peri-implant tissues, including health, height, volume, color, and contours, must be in harmony with the healthy surrounding dentition. The restoration should imitate the natural appearance of the missing dental unit(s) in color, form, texture, size, and optical properties.

Statement C.2
Definition of the Esthetic Zone
Objectively, the esthetic zone was defined as any dentoalveolar segment that is visible upon full smile. Subjectively, the esthetic zone can be defined as any dentoalveolar area of esthetic importance to the patient.

Statement C.3
Measurement of Esthetic Outcomes
The following esthetic-related soft tissue parameters are proposed for use in clinical studies:
- Location of the midfacial mucosal implant margin in relation to the incisal edge or implant shoulder
- Distance between the tip of the papilla and the most apical interproximal contact
- Width of the facial keratinized mucosa
- Assessment of mucosal conditions (e.g., modified Gingival Index, bleeding on probing)
- Subjective measures of esthetic outcomes, such as visual analog scales

Statement C.4
Use of Provisional Restorations
To optimize esthetic treatment outcomes, the use of provisional restorations with adequate emergence profiles is recommended to guide and shape the peri-implant tissue prior to definitive restoration.

Statement C.5
Location of the Implant Shoulder
In most esthetic areas, the implant shoulder is located subgingivally, resulting in a deep interproximal margin. This shoulder location makes seating of the restoration and removal of cement difficult. Therefore, a screw-retained abutment/restoration interface is advisable to minimize these difficulties.

In this volume of the ITI Treatment Guide, the above-listed Consensus Statements will be exemplified by clinical case documentations.

3 Pre-operative Analysis and Prosthetic Treatment Planning in Esthetic Implant Dentistry

W. C. Martin, D. Morton, D. Buser

The goal of risk assessment is to identify patients whose implant therapy carries a high risk of a negative outcome. Therefore, for each patient, a detailed preoperative analysis should be performed to assess the individual risk profile and the level of difficulty of the planned therapy.

Consensus Statement B.1
Planning and Execution:
Implant therapy in the anterior maxilla is considered an advanced or complex procedure and requires comprehensive preoperative planning and precise surgical execution based on a restoration-driven approach.

Consensus Statement B.2
Patient Selection:
Appropriate patient selection is essential in achieving esthetic treatment outcomes. Treatment of high-risk patients identified through site analysis and a general risk assessment (medical status, periodontal susceptibility, smoking, and other risks) should be undertaken with caution, since esthetic results are less consistent.

The initial examination of the patient requiring dental implants in the anterior maxilla should commence with a general treatment risk assessment. Risk assessment in the anterior maxilla of potential implant patients includes several aspects. The patient's past medical history, current medications, allergies, smoking habits, periodontal status and occlusal function should be examined (Buser and coworkers, 2004). Table 1 lists the superordinate, general risk factors in implant patients:

With regard to implant success, high-risk patients should be informed of the challenges associated with the treatment. Alternative restorative methods should be duly considered before planning for dental implant therapy. Patients who qualify for surgical implant procedures from a medical point of view and whose esthetic demands are high should always undergo a detailed examination not only of the edentulous space, but also of the supporting hard and soft tissues. Adjacent teeth, periodontal support, and existing hard and soft tissues are all critical factors when planning for a predictable esthetic result. Together, these factors constitute an assessment of esthetic risk.

In simple terms, the esthetic quality of implant-supported restorations should not differ from that of restorations supported by teeth. They should be in harmony with perioral facial structures, be associated with a healthy surrounding dentition and represent a successful imitation of the missing tooth or teeth with regard to color, form, texture, size, and optical properties (Belser and coworkers, 2004). Achieving such an outcome presupposes a clear understanding of dental esthetics and general esthetic principles, and depends on the treatment team developing an acute diagnostic acumen.

Consensus Statement C.1
Standards for an Esthetic Fixed Implant
Restoration:
An esthetic implant prosthesis was defined as one that is in harmony with the peri-oral facial structures of the patient. The esthetic peri-implant tissues, including health, height, volume, color, and contours, must be in harmony with the healthy surrounding dentition. The restoration should imitate the natural appearance of the missing dental unit(s) in color, form, texture, size, and optical properties.

Table 1 Risk factors in candidates for implant therapy (Buser and coworkers, 2004)

General Risk Factors in Candidates for Implant Therapy	
Risk Factor	Remarks
Medical	• Severe bone disease causing impaired bone healing • Immunologic diseases • Medication with steroids • Uncontrolled diabetes mellitus • Irradiated bone • Others
Periodontal	• Active periodontal disease • History of refractory periodontitis • Genetic disposition
Oral Hygiene/Compliance	• Home care measured by gingival indices • Personality, intellectual aspects
Occlusion	• Bruxism

3.1 Diagnostic Factors for Esthetic Risk Assessment

Diagnostic factors of significance to the pre-treatment examination of the esthetic risk to the treatment outcome include:

1. Patient's treatment expectations
2. Patient's smoking habits
3. Height of the lip line on smiling
4. Gingival biotype in the treatment area
5. Shape of the missing and surrounding teeth
6. Infection at the implant site and bone level at adjacent teeth
7. Restorative status of the teeth adjacent to the edentulous space
8. Character of the edentulous space
9. Width of the hard and soft tissues in the edentulous space
10. Height of the hard and soft tissues in the edentulous space

These criteria can be used to create an *Esthetic Risk Profile* that will help the clinician and patient determine the potential of achieving esthetic results through dental implant therapy.

3.1.1 The Patient's Treatment Expectations

The recent rise in public awareness of the benefits of dental implant therapy has had both positive and negative effects on daily clinical practice. We benefit from the increasing numbers of patients who desire dental implant treatment, but most patients are unaware of what the process entails. Access to the Internet has helped educate patients on how dental implants are used to replace missing teeth. Unfortunately, this education may lead to unrealistic expectations that the treatment team cannot attain. During the consultation visit, it is imperative to determine the patient's ultimate desires. Discussion of the oral rehabilitation project should focus on three aspects: form, function, and esthetics (Garber and coworkers, 1995; Morton and coworkers, 2004). Reviewing these areas with the patient may help generate an initial risk profile for the esthetic outcome and patient acceptance.

Form

Can the edentulous span be restored at all? An evaluation of the restorative space in relationship to adjacent or contralateral teeth will determine if orthodontic or restorative procedures are necessary before or along with implant therapy (Figs 1a, b). Visualizing the planned restoration will also provide information on the available hard and soft-tissue support, whether deficient, adequate, or excessive. Accepted dental procedures, including diagnostic wax-ups and photographs, are important to this visualization.

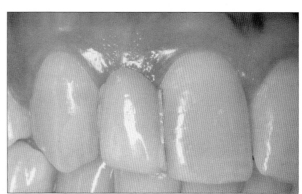

Fig 1a   Pre-treatment examination. Too little restorative space for a dental implant at site 12.

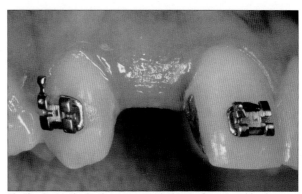

Fig 1b   Post-orthodontic treatment. Ideal space for a dental implant and restoration.

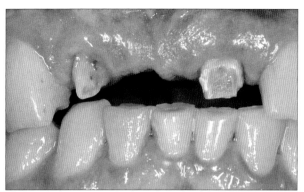

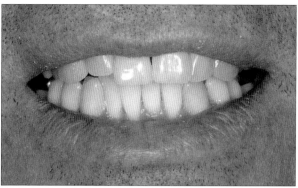

Fig 2   Pre-treatment examination. A lack of available interocclusal space for restoration using dental implants. Treatment of the opposing dentition may be required to achieve long-term implant success.

Fig 3   Low lip line.

Function

An occlusal evaluation is necessary to incorporate the implant-supported restoration into a harmonious and functional environment. In the case of long-standing edentulism, supereruption of the opposing dentition into the free space may make restoration of the implant(s) difficult (Fig 2).

Diagnostic wax-ups help establish a plan for modifying the positions of those teeth and will often be a mandatory component of pre-treatment esthetic analysis.

Esthetics

What are the patient's esthetic expectations? And are they realistic? A detailed discussion with the patient concerning the potential outcome may help avoid disappointing outcomes for patients with high esthetic expectations. Such patients should be considered "high esthetic risks."

> **Consensus Statement C.2**
> **Definition of the Esthetic Zone:**
> Objectively, the esthetic zone was defined as any dentoalveolar segment that is visible upon full smile. Subjectively, the esthetic zone can be defined as any dentoalveolar area of esthetic importance to the patient.

3.1.2   Patient's Smoking Habits

When determining the potential for the esthetic success of a given course of implant treatment, potential complications secondary to the local and general factors should also be considered. Smoking habits may have deleterious effects on grafting procedures, implant integration, or long-term peri-implant tissue health (Buser and coworkers, 2004). Several clinical studies have shown smoking to have a negative impact on the short-term and long-term integration of dental implants (Bain and Moy, 1993; DeBruyn and Collaert, 1994; Lambert and coworkers, 2000; Wallace, 2000). Patients who smoke should be educated on or directed to cessation programs before implant therapy is initiated. Heavy smokers (>10 cig/d) should be considered "high esthetic risks."

3.1.3   Height of the Lip Line on Smiling

The lip line is associated with the amount of tooth substance and supporting tissues visible when the patient chews, speaks, or smiles.

Low Lip Line

Patients who exhibit a low lip line display a predominance of mandibular teeth or an equal mix of maxillary and mandibular teeth. For these patients, the quality of the esthetic outcome is related mostly to the appearance of the incisal half of the maxillary teeth (Fig 3).

Here the "esthetic risk" is reduced as the lips effectively mask suboptimal outcomes associated with the appearance of the gingival tissues, tooth proportions, and the apical aspects of the restoration.

The diagnostic waxup helped select the right type of restoration and the right type of abutment.

In this case, the clinical situation did not allow for a screw-retained restoration due to the relatively far palatal position of the incisal edges of the central incisors. To simplify the lab procedure by using the same materials for the reconstruction of both the natural tooth and the implant, it was decided to use a ceramic blank (synOcta In-Ceram blank, material: VITA In-Ceram ZIRCONIA) on the implant.

A silicone key was produced to capture the tooth shapes from the waxup and used for evaluation of the ideal abutment dimensions (Fig 41).

After shaping the In-Ceram blank, special attention was paid to checking the precise dimensions of its marginal aspect and the position of the future cement line, and the respective minimal dimensions necessary for optimum mechanical stability (Fig 42).

A check of the incisal edge positions revealed that the In-Ceram blank's incisal edge portion was located too far labially (Fig 43) and needed to be corrected (Fig 44). Note the special blue anodized occlusal screw used to tighten the In-Ceram blank on the synOcta abutment.

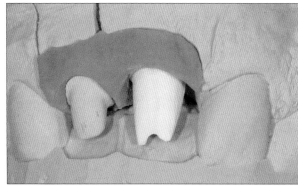

Fig 41   Silicone key representing the diagnostic waxup used to determine and control the shape and form of the individual abutment.

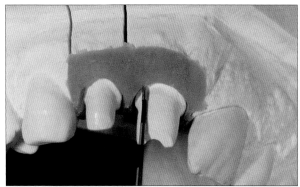

Fig 42   Prospective crown margin, ideally placed 1 to 2 mm subgingivally.

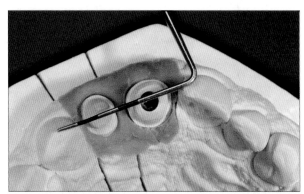

Fig 43   The incisal edge of the In-Ceram blank was located too far labially; this had to be corrected.

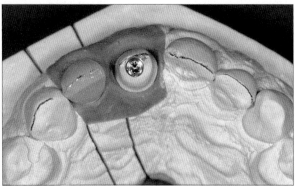

Fig 44   The corrected In-Ceram blank's incisal edge portion.

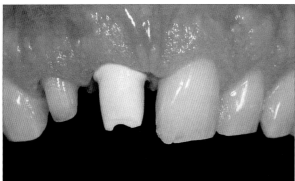

Fig 45   Abutment try-in, checking the form and position of the preparation margin. Adjustments can be performed directly in the mouth with a high-speed angled handpiece or by marking the correct position with a pen.

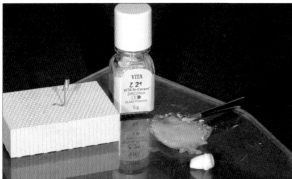

Fig 46   Glass powder mixed with distilled water for application to the blank.

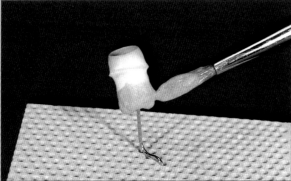

Fig 47   Infiltration of the blank in the dental lab.

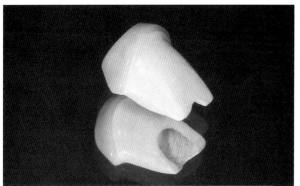

Fig 48   Final glass-infiltrated abutment with stained cervical aspect.

At try-in seven months after implantation and four months after installation of the first temporary abutment, the synOcta In-Ceram blank was carefully screw-tightened onto the synOcta abutment by hand. Again, special attention was paid to the evaluation of the position of the mucosal margin in relation to the preparation margin of the blank and its cervical, submucosal aspect (Fig 45). To ensure optimal cement removal, the cement line should be placed 1 – 2 mm submucosally.

In order to be able to adapt the shape of the blank based on the outcome of the try-in, the blank was tried in its porously sintered, non-infiltrated state and infiltrated after the chairside try-in session (Fig 46, 47).

After the infiltration process that gave the porously sintered, chalky blank its final strength and stability, the cervical portion was stained according to the dentine color of neighboring tooth 12 (Fig 48).

R. Jung

After the first bake, the shape and fit of the all-ceramic crowns were checked on the model (Fig 49).

After the second bake, the crowns integrated harmoniously with the existing dentition (Fig 50). Note the natural color of the mucosa and the harmonious line of the marginal gingiva and mucosa.

When the result of the try-in in the patient's mouth was found to be acceptable, the all-ceramic crowns were finalized in the dental lab (Figs 51, 52)

The crowns were etched with hydrofluoric acid in the dental lab. Silane was applied at chairside.

The all-ceramic crown for the implant superstructure in position 11 perfectly matched the individually stained cervical portion of the In-Ceram blank and precisely fit on top of it (Fig 53).

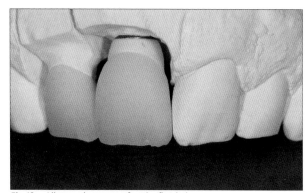

Fig 49   All-ceramic crowns after the first bake.

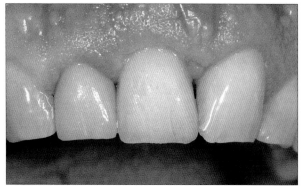

Fig 50   Try-in of the crowns after the second bake.

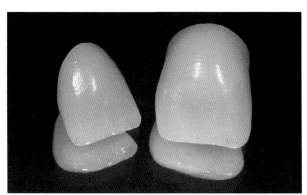

Fig 51   Final glass-ceramic crowns.

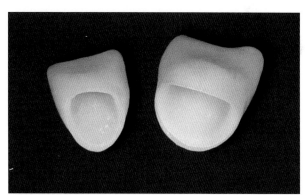

Fig 52   Final glass-ceramic crowns before cementation.

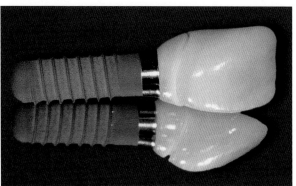

Fig 53   Final crown on the individualized In-Ceram blank.

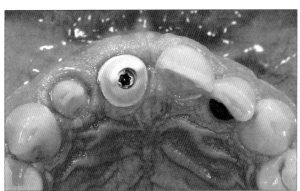

Fig 54 Final blank, placed on the synOcta abutment with the blue an-odized occlusal screw tightened to 15 Ncm .

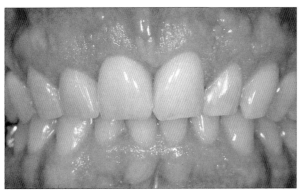

Fig 55 After adhesive cementation of the two crowns, harmonious integration into the natural dentition.

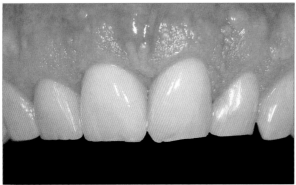

Fig 56 Final implant-supported all-ceramic crown 11 and tooth-supported all-ceramic crown 12.

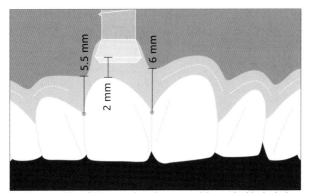

Fig 57 A stable soft-tissue level can be expected due to the ideal relations of bone crest, implant shoulder, and contact points.

The In-Ceram blank was screwed in place on the synOcta abutment with the blue anodized occlusal screw tightened to 15 Ncm (Fig 54).

The final implant-supported superstructure integrated into the natural dentition harmoniously. The shape of the crown on tooth 12 as well as the shape of the implant-supported crown at site 11 perfectly matched the shape, texture, and size of the corresponding contralateral natural teeth. The lines of the marginal gingiva and mucosa were symmetrical. The gingival and mucosal colors were natural and matched that of the rest of the gingiva. The papillae filled the interdental spaces completely, without leaving "black triangles" (Figs 55, 56)

The incisal edges were symmetrical to those of the contralateral natural teeth (Fig 56). At this point, the treatment could be considered an esthetic success.

The distance between the contact points and marginal bone crest levels on the mesial and distal of the implant did not exceed 5 mm (Fig 57). Therefore, one would expect the soft-tissue level to remain stable and no "black triangles" to develop in the interdental spaces over time.

At full smile, the patient presented an esthetically pleasing row of maxillary teeth. The implant-supported superstructure harmoniously blends in with the row of natural teeth (Fig 58).

The periapical radiograph after installation of the superstructure confirmed its gap-free seating on the implant shoulder (Fig 59).

The three-year follow-up photographs (Figs 60 – 61) demonstrate a stable esthetic treatment outcome.

The three-year follow-up periapical radiograph demonstrated stable bone levels around the implant (Fig 62).

Acknowledgment

Laboratory Procedures
Master Dental Technician Ana Suter – University of Zurich, Switzerland, Clinic for Dental Crown and Bridge Prosthetics, Partial Prosthetics, and Dental Material Science

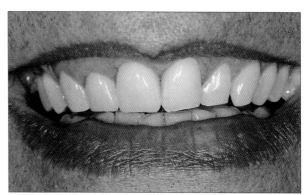

Fig 58   Full smile with final restorations.

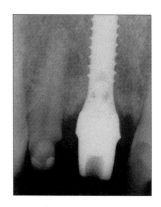

Fig 59   Radiograph before cementation. Gap-free seating of the superstructure on the implant shoulder.

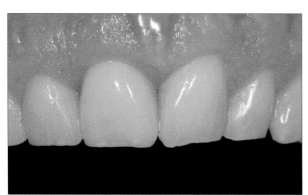

Fig 60   Buccal view three years after implant insertion.

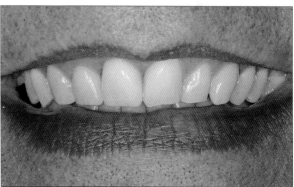

Fig 61   Smile three years after implant insertion.

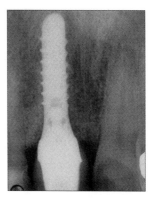

Fig 62   Periapical radiograph three years after implant insertion.

4.7 Replacement of an Upper Right Central Incisor with a Regular Neck Implant, Restored with an All-Ceramic Crown, Cemented

W. C. Martin

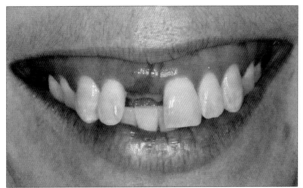

Fig 1   At full smile, the patient presented with a high lip line exposing full clinical crowns, papillae, and gingival tissues.

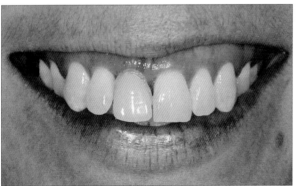

Fig 2   With the interim prosthesis in place, it was evident that teeth 13 and 12 were malpositioned.

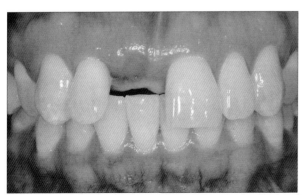

Fig 3   Retracted view showing the excessive overbite and malpositioning of teeth 13 and 12 .

A healthy 32-year-old female patient presented for a consultation on treatment options to restore her missing central incisor 11 (Fig 1).

She reported of a recent sporting accident in which she had lost part of her tooth. The remaining tooth structure and root had been removed by a local periodontist, followed by a socket-preservation procedure. She was unaware of current treatment options to replace her missing tooth and wanted to explore the most esthetic and functional options available. A brief consultation showed that the patient was not interested in orthognathic procedures to address her maxillary overbite, nor in any alternative procedures to lower her high lip line. With her interim prosthesis in place, an evaluation of her smile highlighted several malpositioned teeth surrounding tooth 11. Comparing the maxillary canines, it was evident that tooth 13 was rotated. Comparison of the lateral incisors revealed that tooth 12 had a flared appearance (Fig 2). A detailed examination of the teeth and periodontium adjacent to the edentulous space was performed to assess the esthetic risk for implant therapy.

An occlusal evaluation revealed coincident maxillary and mandibular midlines, mutually protected occlusion, and approximately 75% overbite (Fig 3).

The gingival biotype was thin with moderately scalloped papillae, thin tissue, broad keratinized tissue, and slightly tapered teeth (Fig 4). Pontic tooth 11 was ovate in shape, indicating adequate facial tissue height in the edentulous space. A soft-tissue examination revealed a deficiency in papillary support on the mesiofacial aspect of teeth 12 and 21. Probing depths at teeth 12 and 21 were 2 mm palatally, 2 mm interproximally, and 1 mm facially. It was also apparent that an adequate horizontal tissue thickness existed, allowing for good "root-form" emergence of the proposed implant restoration (Fig 5).

The examination of the periapical radiograph revealed the presence of borderline space (6.5 mm) between the roots of the adjacent teeth. Good interproximal bone support is evident on the teeth adjacent to the edentulous space (Fig 6).

After the consultation, the data obtained were compiled for the esthetic risk-assessment table (Table 1).

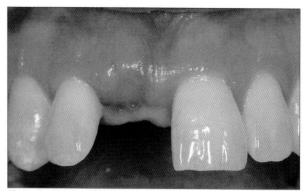

Fig 4   Frontal view of moderately tapered teeth, harmonious gingival margins, and papillary deficiencies on the mesiofacial aspect of teeth 12 and 21.

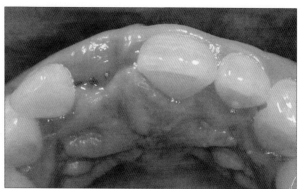

Fig 5   Occlusal view highlighting good horizontal ridge support in the edentulous space.

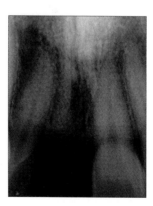

Fig 6   Periapical radiograph at site 11. Interproximal space at mid-root level is 6.5 mm, alveolar crest height 5 mm from the desired contact point.

Table 1   The patient's individual esthetic risk profile.

Esthetic Risk Factors	Low	Medium	High
Medical status	Healthy and cooperative patient and intact immune system		Reduced immune system
Smoking habit	Non-smoker	Light smoker (< 10 cig/d)	Heavy smoker (≥ 10 cig/d)
Patient's esthetic expectations	Low	Medium	High
Lip line	Low	Medium	High
Gingival biotype	Low scalloped, thick	Medium scalloped, medium thick	High scalloped, thin
Shape of tooth crowns	Rectangular		Triangular
Infection at implant site	None	Chronic	Acute
Bone level at adjacent teeth	≤ 5 mm to contact point	5.5 to 6.5 mm to contact point	≥ 7 mm to contact point
Restorative status of neighboring teeth	Virgin		Restored
Width of edentulous span	1 tooth (≥ 7 mm)	1 tooth (< 7 mm)	2 teeth or more
Soft-tissue anatomy	Intact soft tissue		Soft-tissue defects
Bone anatomy of alveolar crest	Alveolar crest without bone deficiency	Horizontal bone deficiency	Vertical bone deficiency

Taking into consideration the patient's restorative desires, high lip line, thin-gingiva biotype, and deficiencies in papillae adjacent to site 11, multiple treatment options were considered. When the pros and cons of fixed treatment options were provided, the patient insisted on the implant option, as it would not rely on support from the adjacent teeth. The overall esthetic risk for this treatment is high. This indicates that the potential for an esthetic result to be achieved with an implant-supported restoration, as based on the ITI Consensus Statements (Belser and coworkers, 2004), is low. With this guarded diagnosis, a comprehensive treatment plan was generated to treat the edentulous site with a team approach. All of the potential outcomes were reviewed with the patient before proceeding with the treatment. Esthetic risks associated with the procedure ranged from: lack of papillary support adjacent to the dental implant restoration, discolored mucosal tissue facial to the implant, a square restoration to mask an interproximal tissue deficiency, and lack of harmonious tissue margins.

Three phases of treatment were planned:

1. Orthodontics – Would be performed to reduce the vertical overlap and align the canine (13) and lateral (12) into the arch form and to create more space between the roots of teeth 12 and 21.
2. Surgery – Using a restoration-driven approach, placing a Regular Neck (RN), Standard Plus (SP) dental implant.
3. Restorative – A provisional fabricated in addition to a final restoration focusing on form, function and esthetics.

Orthodontic therapy reduced the overbite and rounded out the maxillary arch (Fig 7). A denture tooth was bonded to a bracket and attached to the orthodontic archwire, providing esthetics while tooth movement occurred (Fig 8). Moderate rotational torque was applied to create root space between teeth 12 and 21. Upon completion of the orthodontic treatment, the patient was seen before the removal of the brackets to fabricate a surgical template and to insert the dental implant. Utilizing the brackets to retain the denture tooth after implant surgery and before loading provided a stable and esthetic interim prosthesis.

Prior to surgery, a radiographic template was fabricated to assure proper placement of the dental implant (Fig 9).

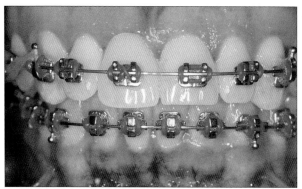

Fig 7   Frontal view showed the improvement in gingival margin relationships and resolution of the excessive overbite as achieved through orthodontic therapy.

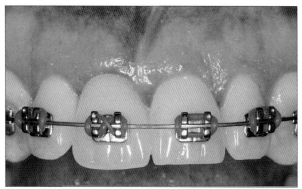

Fig 8   Denture tooth replacing tooth 11 attached to the orthodontic archwire throughout the orthodontic treatment.

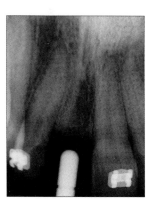

Fig 9   Periapical view with the radiographic template in place.

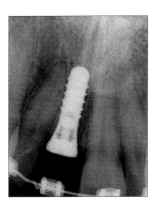

Fig 10   Periapical radiograph after implant placement.

A surgical template was fabricated based upon the results of the radiographic survey and utilized during the surgical procedure. At the surgical visit, a scalloping procedure was done to allow proper vertical placement of the RN SP implant. The vertical positioning template assured ideal coronoapical positioning while template with the drill sleeve was utilized to prepare the osteotomy site. Once the implant had been placed, the vertical depth (shoulder 2 mm apically of the proposed mucosal margin) was confirmed once more before removing the implant mount. After placement of the labially beveled healing cap and suturing, a periapical radiograph was taken (Fig 10).

The denture tooth was adjusted so it did not contact the healing cap when the archwire was in place. The patient was scheduled for a one-week follow-up.

Six weeks after implant placement, the patient was scheduled for a loading visit (Fig 11). At this appointment, a provisional restoration was made that would initiate maturation of the transition zone. Upon removal of the orthodontic archwire, it became evident that the healing cap was semi-submerged (Figs 12a, b).

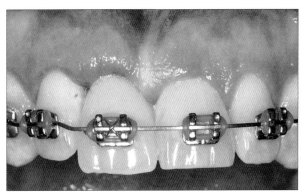

Fig 11   Six weeks after implant placement.

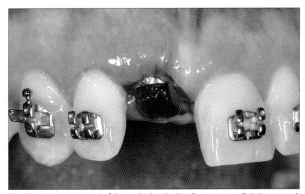

Fig 12a   Upon removal of the archwire, the healing cap was slightly exposed, allowing for access to the implant shoulder with minimal tissue removal.

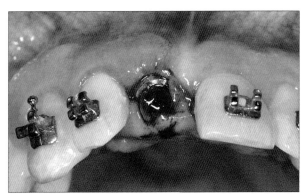

Fig 12b   Occlusal view of the excess tissue that covered the palatal portion of the healing cap.

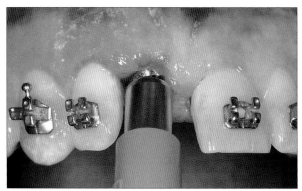

Fig 13a   A 5-mm biopsy tissue punch was used to remove the tissue that covered the healing cap.

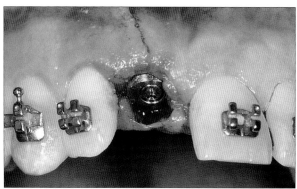

Fig 13b   Upon the removal of the tissue, the healing cap was easily accessible.

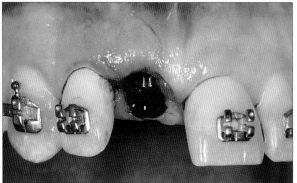

Fig 14a   After removal of the healing cap, the implant was cleaned with an air-water syringe before placing the interim abutment.

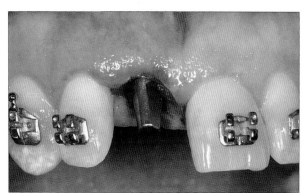

Fig 14b   A 5.5-mm solid abutment was tightened to 15 Ncm to be utilized as an interim abutment.

Excess tissue was located on the palatal surface of the healing cap. Upon examination, it appeared that there was no benefit in keeping the tissue, so a 5-mm biopsy punch was utilized to carefully remove that excess tissue (Figs 13a, b).

Based upon its ease of use, a 5.5-mm solid abutment was used to fabricate the provisional restoration (Figs 14a, b). As reported in the ITI Consensus statements (Belser and coworkers, 2004), when the shoulder of the implant is greater than 3 mm submucosally, a screw-retained machined margin connection is recommended to prevent entrapment of cement. While not in line with the ITI Consensus statements, a solid abutment was utilized due to the implant position (exiting through the incisal edge) and clinician preference. A preformed polycarbonate shell was relined with methylmethacrylate resin to fabricate the provisional restoration (Fig 15).

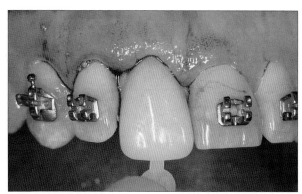

Fig 15   A polycarbonate shell was relined with methylmethacrylate resin over the solid abutment.

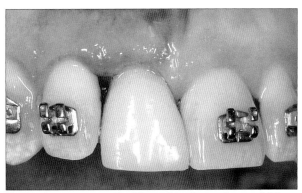

Fig 16   The emergence profile of the provisional restoration was slightly undercontoured in all dimensions to prevent movement of the tissue in an apical direction.

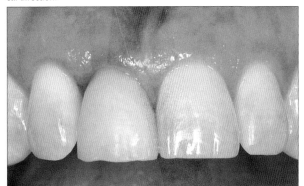

Fig 17   Two weeks post-loading with the provisional restoration.

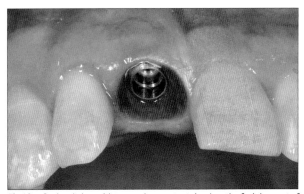

Fig 18   Occlusal view with trapped cement retained on the facial aspect of the implant shoulder.

Once the provisional material had set intraorally, it was removed and placed onto a practice abutment and analog. Using some powder and monomer in dappen dishes and a brush, acrylic resin was added to the provisional to create an emergence profile from the implant shoulder into the oral cavity. Upon placement of the provisional in the mouth, tissue blanching subsided within 10 minutes. The provisional was cemented with temporary cement, and the occlusion was adjusted (Fig 16).

Due to the high esthetic challenge of this treatment, the patient was brought back after two weeks for a follow-up.

At the return visit, a moderate amount of tissue inflammation remained around the facial mucosal margin (Fig 17).

Upon removal of the provisional and abutment, excess cement was located under the facial shoulder of the implant (Fig 18). It was decided at this visit to make a synOcta impression for the fabrication of an indirect provisional that would remove any possibility of cement entrapment by bringing the cement line closer to the tissue surface.

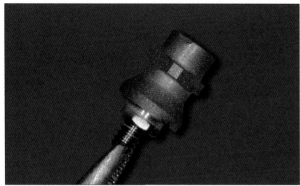

Fig 19a   Modified synOcta post for temporary restorations.

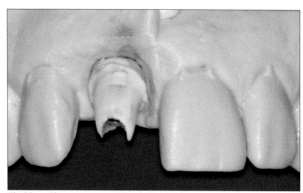

Fig 20a   The custom provisional abutment was modified on the master cast.

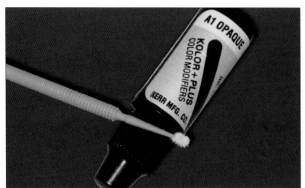

Fig 19b   Kerr Kolor Plus opaque (Kerr).

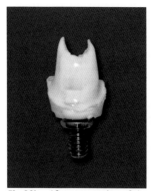

Fig 20b   After preparation of the provisional abutment, facial view.

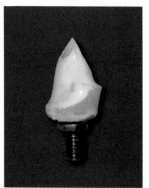

Fig 20c   After preparation of the provisional abutment, lateral view.

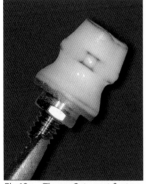

Fig 19c   The synOcta post for temporary restorations after application of the opaque.

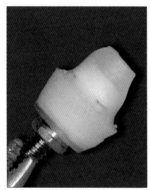

Fig 19d   The synOcta post for temporary restorations built up with a composite resin.

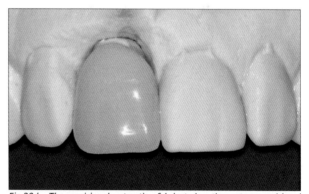

Fig 20d   The provisional restoration fabricated on the custom provisional abutment.

In the laboratory, a synOcta post for temporary restorations was modified to create a custom temporary abutment (Figs 19a-d).

Once fabricated, the custom temporary abutment was placed on the cast and prepared to create restorative margins slightly below the proposed mucosal margin. Upon completion of the preparation, a cementable provisional restoration was fabricated utilizing an acrylic-resin laminate procedure (Figs 20a-d).

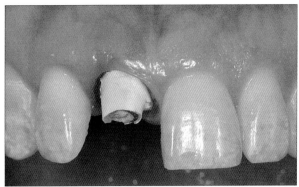

Fig 21a   Facial view of the customized provisional abutment.

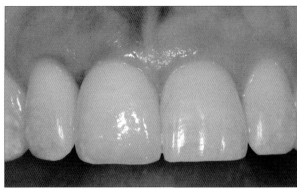

Fig 22a   Four weeks after delivery of the provisional restoration.

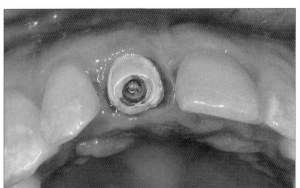

Fig 21b   Occlusal view of the customized provisional abutment.

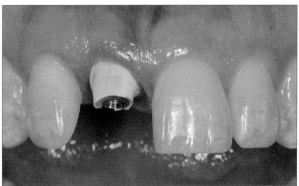

Fig 22b   After removal of the provisional restoration.

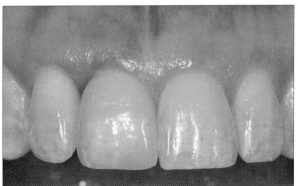

Fig 21c   After cementation of the provisional restoration.

The patient returned to the clinic for insertion of the custom provisional abutment and provisional. After removal of the previous provisional and solid abutment, the custom provisional abutment was tightened to 15 Ncm, and the second provisional with improved emergence profiles was cemented with temporary cement (Figs 21a-c).

The goal of this provisional restoration was to bring the cement line to a clinically accessible location and reduce the potential for continued inflammation on the facial aspect of the implant. The patient was scheduled for a final impression two weeks later.

The maturation of the peri-implant tissue and the reduction in inflammation could be appreciated at the return visit (Figs 22a-b).

The provisional and abutment was removed and the implant was cleansed with air and water, allowing the maturation of the transition zone to be appreciated (Figs 23a-b).

Before the final impression, the shade was taken (Fig 24).

With a synOcta impression cap in place, the lack of peri-implant tissue support was evident in the interproximal areas (Fig 25). Therefore, the fabrication of a custom impression cap would allow vital information of the transition zone to be transferred to the technician to enhance the final emergence of the definitive abutment and restoration. At chairside, the provisional abutment and crown were utilized to modify the impression cap (Figs 26 a-f).

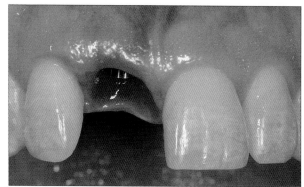

Fig 23a   Upon removal of the provisional abutment, the maturation of the transition zone was noticeable.

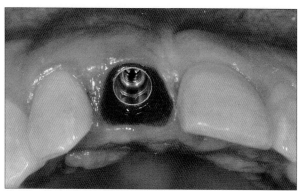

Fig 23b   Occlusal view of tooth 11, highlighting the transition zone.

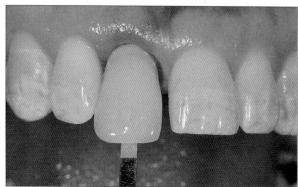

Fig 24   Shade selection before making the final impression.

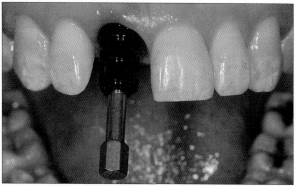

Fig 25   Facial view of an unmodified synOcta impression cap. Note the lack of interproximal tissue support.

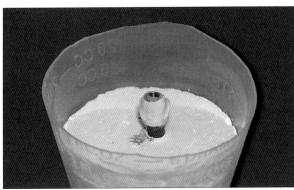

Fig 26a   Custom impression cap fabrication. Provisional abutment on the synOcta analog.

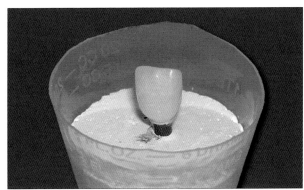

Fig 26b   Custom impression cap fabrication. Provisional on the abutment.

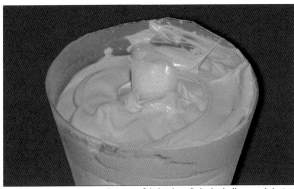

Fig 26c   Custom impression cap fabrication. Polyvinyl siloxane injected against the provisional.

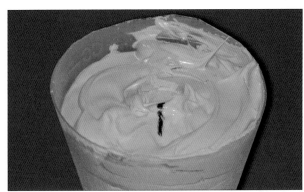

Fig 26d   Custom impression cap fabrication. Once set, the provisional and the abutment were removed.

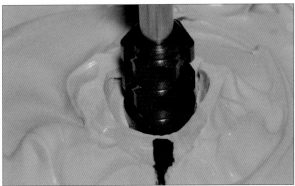

Fig 26e   Custom impression cap fabrication. synOcta impression cap (with handle) on the analog.

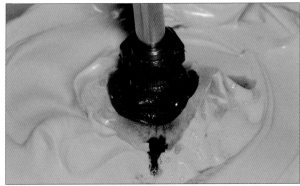

Fig 26f   Custom impression cap fabrication. A flowable resin (GC Pattern Resin, GC America) in the void around the impression cap.

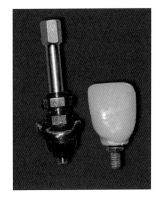

Fig 27   Custom impression cap fabrication. Emergence of the customized impression cap similar to the provisional restoration.

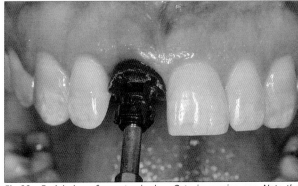

Fig 28   Facial view of a customized synOcta impression cap. Note the added support of interproximal tissue.

Upon completion of the modification to the impression cap, comparison with the provisional revealed similar emergence profiles of the implant shoulder (Fig 27).

With the custom impression cap in place, a polyvinyl siloxane impression was taken (Fig 28).

In the laboratory, an implant analog was placed into the impression coping and soft-tissue analog material was injected around the customized impression post and allowed to set (Figs 29a-b).

A low-expansion die stone was poured into the final impression and allowed to set. Upon removal, the transition zone was clearly seen on the master cast (Fig 30).

A synOcta gold abutment was selected as the definitive abutment for this case (Fig 31).

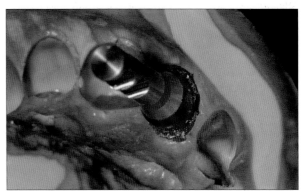

Fig 29a   Laboratory analog attached to the customized impression cap.

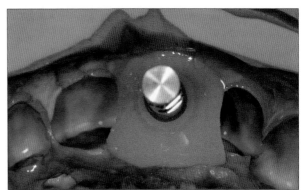

Fig 29b   Soft-tissue analog (Gingitech, Ivolcar) placed around the analog and customized impression cap.

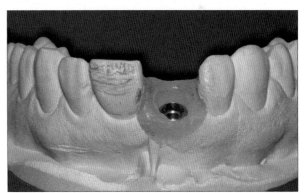

Fig 30   Master cast. Note the duplication of the clinical transition zone in the soft-tissue analog.

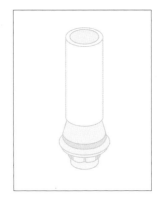

Fig 31
The synOcta gold abutment.

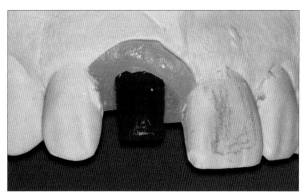

Fig 32a   Facial view of the wax buildup on the synOcta gold abutment.

Due to the thin soft tissues, a ceramic-modified surface was planned for the definitive custom abutment to prevent any submucosal reflection of metal. Once the abutment had been placed onto the master cast, it was modified to provide space for the ceramic material. Wax was then applied to the surface to cast an oxidizable alloy onto the abutment to allow for ceramic application (Figs 32a-d).

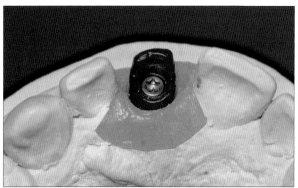

Fig 32b   Occlusal view of the wax buildup on the synOcta gold abutment.

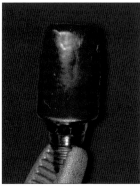

Fig 32c   Facial view of the waxup.

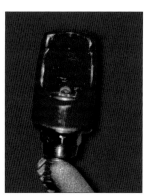

Fig 32d   Palatal view of the waxup.

After the abutment was cast, it was then opaqued, followed by a ceramic buildup designed to support the soft-tissue analog and maintain a submucosal margin position (Figs 33a-c).

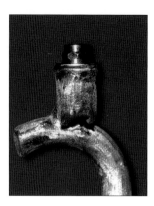

Fig 33a   Casting before removal of the sprue.

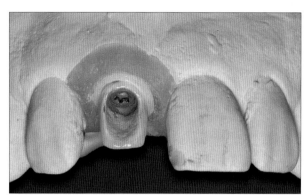

Fig 33b   Frontal view of the synOcta gold abutment customized with ceramics.

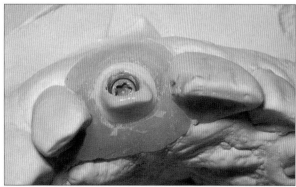

Fig 33c   Palatal view of the synOcta gold abutment customized with ceramics.

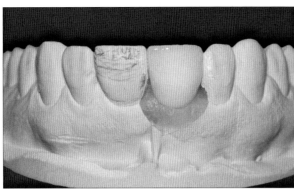

Fig 34   The In-Ceram restoration on the customized abutment.

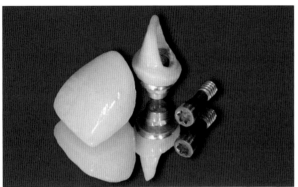

Fig 35a   Final restoration and abutment returned from the laboratory.

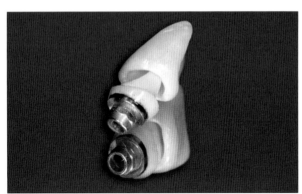

Fig 35b   Exploded view of the relationship between the crown and abutment.

Upon completion of the customized abutment, an all-ceramic In-Ceram crown was fabricated with a 360° ceramic butt-joint margin (Fig 34).

The custom abutment and crown were returned to the clinic for delivery to the patient (Figs 35a-b).

At the delivery visit four weeks after impression-taking, the provisional restoration and abutment were removed (Fig 36). The implant was irrigated with the air-water syringe before placement of the customized abutment. Once the fit and shade of the final restoration had been confirmed, the abutment screw was tightened to 35 Ncm (Figs 37a-c).

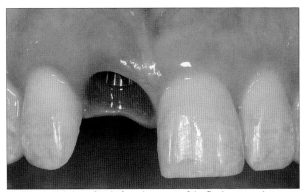

Fig 36   Facial view of 11 before placement of the final custom abutment.

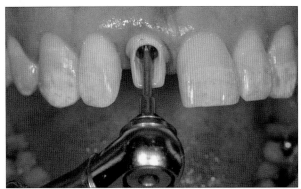

Fig 37a   Tightening of the custom abutment to 35 Ncm using the ratchet with torque control device.

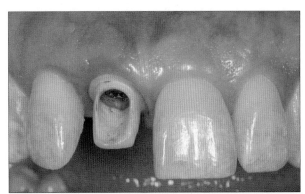

Fig 37b   Facial view of the custom abutment in place. Note the submucosal margins, accessible for cement cleanup.

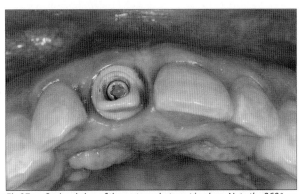

Fig 37c   Occlusal view of the custom abutment in place. Note the 360° ceramic butt margin.

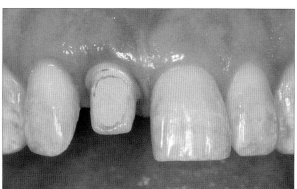

Fig 38   Cotton and Cavit placed to seal access to the abutment screw.

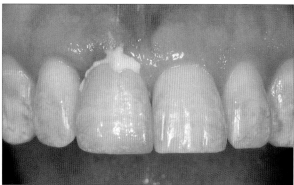

Fig 39   After cementation of the restoration, allowing for accessible cement cleanup.

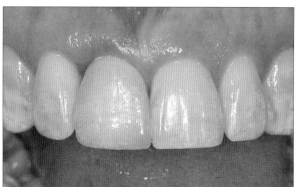

Fig 40a   After delivery of the In-Ceram crown for tooth 11.

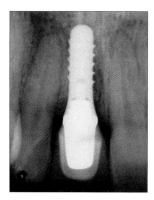

Fig 40b   Periapical radiograph after delivery.

The screw access hole was covered with a cotton pellet and sealed with Cavit (3M Espe) (Fig 38). The final restoration was cemented with permanent cement. Excess cement was removed after setting (Fig 39).

The occlusion was adjusted to a light shim-stock pull. Adjustments to the ceramic surface were followed by polishing with diamond-impregnated disks that help to create a glaze-like surface on the ceramic. A periapical radiograph was taken and the patient was scheduled for a 3-week follow-up (Figs 40a-b).

At the 3-week visit, the peri-implant tissues were examined for residual cement and the occlusion checked. Oral hygiene procedures were reviewed with the patient. After the visit, the patient was scheduled for yearly maintenance procedures.

The patient was seen after her maintenance visit for a follow-up after one year (Figs 41a-c).

Acknowledgments

Orthodontic Procedures
Dr. Dawn Martin – J & M Orthodontics, Gainesville, Florida, USA

Surgical Procedures
Dr. Caleb King – Private Practice, Gainesville, Florida, USA

Laboratory Procedures
Mitchell Jim – M & M Dental Laboratory, Gainesville, Florida, USA

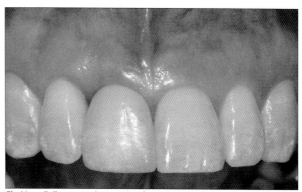

Fig 41a   Follow-up twelve months after delivery. The harmonious gingival margins, tooth positions, and interproximal tissue support can be appreciated.

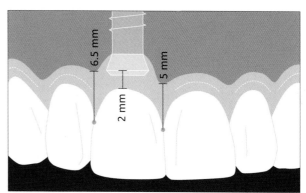

Fig 41b   A stable esthetic treatment outcome due to correct three-dimensional implant placement.

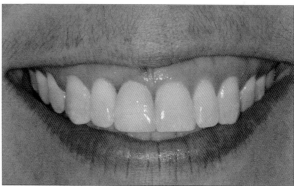

Fig 41c   Follow-up twelve months after delivery, full smile.

4.8 Replacement of an Upper Left Central Incisor with a Regular Neck Implant, Restored with a Ceramo-Metal Crown, Transocclusally Screw-Retained

R. Jung

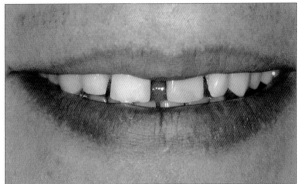

Fig 1 The slight smile presents a harmonious relation between the course of the incisor edges and the lower lips.

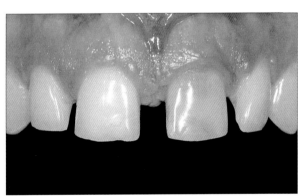

Fig 2 The tissue biotype was medium thick with a medium scallop.

The 23-old-male patient, a light smoker (less than five cigarettes per day), presented with a non-vital and discolored tooth 21 (Fig 1). The patient was in good general health, and his medical history was without significant findings. He suffered from pain originating from mobile tooth 21. Because of the discoloration of tooth 21, the patient asked to have his esthetic appearance improved. Tooth 21 had been endodontically treated after trauma, and an apicoectomy had been performed.

At full smile, the patient had a medium smile line, exposing the full teeth and part of the gingiva.

The patient's gingival biotype was medium thick, with a sufficiently thick band of attached keratinized gingiva (Fig 2). The tissue was free of recessions or other defects.

The line of the gingival margin and the line of the incisal edges were harmonious.

In general, a quadrangular tooth shape has the advantage of reducing the esthetic risk due to the long interproximal contact areas that help compensate for black triangles. In a diastema case like this, however, a lack of interproximal tissue cannot be compensated for by prosthetic treatment. Orthodontic treatment and increasing the mesiodistal tooth diameters could help lower the esthetic risk. The patient was asked if he wanted to undergo orthodontic therapy to re-align his teeth and to increase the mesiodistal diameter of the incisors using either composite or ceramic veneers. The patient's desire was to keep his characteristic appearance. He asked for replacement of tooth 21 only, without any additional orthodontic or prosthetic therapy.

As Figure 3 demonstrates, the labial contours of the alveolar arch were maintained by tooth 21.

Clinical probing of tooth 21 revealed a mesial pocket depth of 7 mm and a buccal pocket depth of 10 mm.

Radiologically, a radiolucency mesially of tooth 21 could be detected. These findings are symptomatic of a root fracture of the endodontically treated tooth 21, status after apicoectomy (Fig 4).

Looking at the adjacent teeth, the interproximal bone levels were judged to be sufficiently well maintained for adequate soft-tissue support after implant therapy (Fig 5).

Due to the increased probing depth at the buccal aspect of tooth 21, a lack of buccal bone lamina had to be expected. Hence, the possibility of a major bone defect had to be considered, which would necessitate bone augmentation with or without simultaneous implant placement.

Based upon the data collected during the clinical and radiological examination, the patient's esthetic risk-profile analysis was as follows (Table 1):

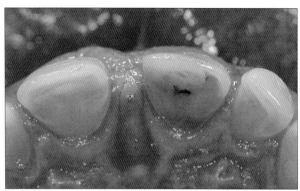

Fig 3   Occlusal view of the incisors.

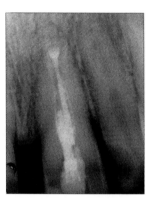

Fig 4   Periapical radiograph showing a mesial radiolucency and the status after apicoectomy.

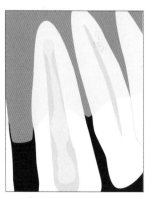

Fig 5   Evaluating the interproximal bone levels around the teeth adjacent to the future implant site is important for the evaluation of the esthetic risk.

Table 1   The patient's individual esthetic risk profile.

Esthetic Risk Factors	Low	Medium	High
Medical status	Healthy and cooperative patient, intact immune system		Reduced immune system
Smoking habit	Non-smoker	Light smoker (< 10 cig/d)	Heavy smoker (> 10 cig/d)
Patient's esthetic expectations	Low	Medium	High
Lip line	Low	Medium	High
Gingival biotype	Low scalloped, thick	Medium scalloped, medium thick	High scalloped, thin
Shape of tooth crowns	Rectangular		Triangular
Infection at implant site	None	Chronic	Acute
Bone level at adjacent teeth	≤ 5 mm to contact point	5.5 to 6.5 mm to contact point	≥ 7 mm to contact point
Restorative status of neighboring teeth	Virgin		Restored
Width of edentulous span	1 tooth (≥ 7 mm)	1 tooth (< 7 mm)	2 teeth or more
Soft-tissue anatomy	Intact soft tissue		Soft-tissue defects
Bone anatomy of alveolar crest	Alveolar crest without bone deficiency	Horizontal bone deficiency	Vertical bone deficiency

The diastema situation in combination with the expected large bone defect made this a medium to high risk case.

The pre-extraction orthopantomograph showed sufficient bone thickness apically of tooth 21. It also showed that teeth 11 and 22 and their periodontal structures were healthy. The mesiodistal width of the future implant site was sufficient (Fig 6).

Because of the expected major bone-augmentation procedure, a thick, mature mucosa at the prospective implant site was desirable. A healing period of six to eight weeks after tooth extraction (Type 2 implant placement, Hämmerle and coworkers, 2004) was chosen to allow for soft tissue healing.

Either a primary bone-augmentation procedure or implant placement with simultaneous bone augmentation could be performed at the time of reopening. The decision was based on the ability of stabilizing the implant in the proper prosthetic position.

The site was reopened eight weeks after extraction. An osseous defect with the expected large buccal dehiscence was present (Fig 7).

The incisal view shows the full extent of the horizontal bone defect (Fig 8).

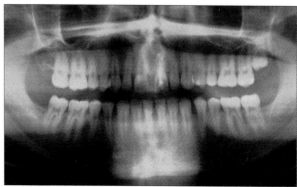

Fig 6   The pre-extraction orthopantomograph was used for pre-implantation diagnostics and treatment planning.

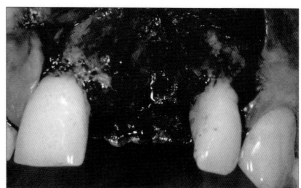

Fig 7   A large buccal dehiscence at reopening, eight weeks after extraction.

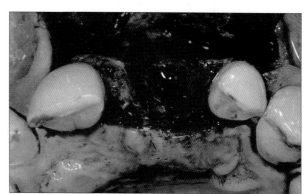

Fig 8   The bone defect at the future implant site had a large horizontal component.

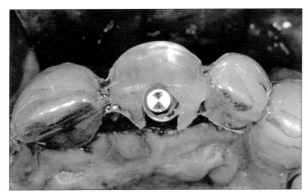

Fig 9   The surgical template facilitated ideal three-dimensional, prosthetically driven implant placement.

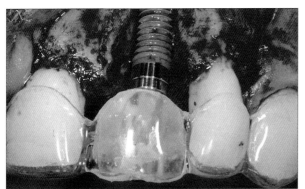

Fig 10   The implant was to be located about 2 mm apically of the border of the surgical template representing the future soft-tissue margin of the implant crown.

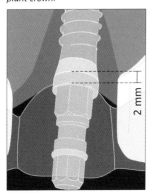

Fig 11   A surgical template helping to visualize the future soft-tissue margin, ideally located about 2 mm coronally of the implant shoulder.

To facilitate an ideal three-dimensional implant placement in accordance with the planned future position of the implant-supported crown, a surgical template was used for correct implant placement (Figs 9, 10).

It is important, especially in diastema situations, to ensure implementation of the pre-operative diagnostics and treatment planning during surgery. The use of a surgical template for implant placement is therefore highly recommended in these cases.

The surgical template not only ensured the correct orofacial implant position, but it also determined the correct coronoapical position (Figs 10, 11).

In its ideal coronoapical position, the implant shoulder is located about 2 mm apically of the future soft-tissue margin at the implant-supported crown, imitated by the apical border of the template (Fig 11).

The situation after removal of the surgical template showed the ideal three-dimensional position of the implant (Tapered Effect (TE) implant, endosseous Ø 4.1 mm, Regular Neck, Ø 4.8 mm) achieved despite the large bone defect (Figs 12, 13). Especially in large bone defects, the increased thread pitch of the TE implant facilitates primary stability.

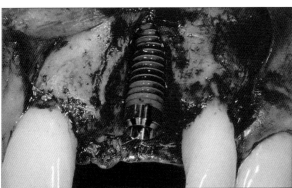

Fig 12   Implant in its ideal coronoapical position.

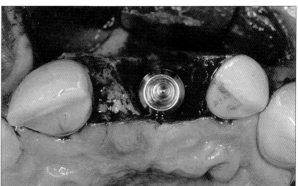

Fig 13   Ideal mesiodistal and orofacial implant positions.

Because sufficient apical bone volume was available, the implant could be placed easily and it attained good primary stability. The site could thus be treated in a simultaneous approach, combining implant placement and bone augmentation. Membranes with improved mechanical properties have advantages for the regeneration of large bone defects in that they predictably re-establish the bone contour that was lost. For large defects, the concept for bone regeneration therefore includes the use of a titanium-reinforced membrane together with autogenous bone and grafting material.

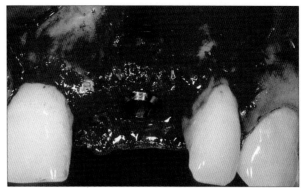

Fig 14   Applying autogenous bone around the implant shoulder.

The autogenous bone, harvested from the osteotomy site and the anterior nasal spine, was applied to the implant neck portion (Fig 14).

The osseous defect was completely filled with grafting material.

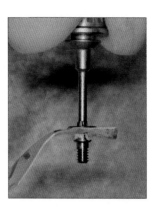

The augmentation site was subsequently covered with a titanium-reinforced e-PTFE membrane in order to stabilize the augmentation site and to preserve the desired contour.

To prevent dislocation of the membrane, it was fixed with pins as well as the implant's closure screw (Figs 15, 16).

Fig 15   Perforating the membrane for insertion of the closure screw.

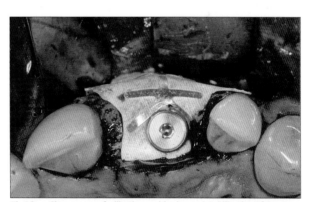

Fig 16a   Closure screw facilitating positioning and stabilization of the membrane.

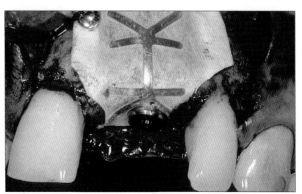

Fig 16b   Additional pins ensuring stable fixation of the membrane.

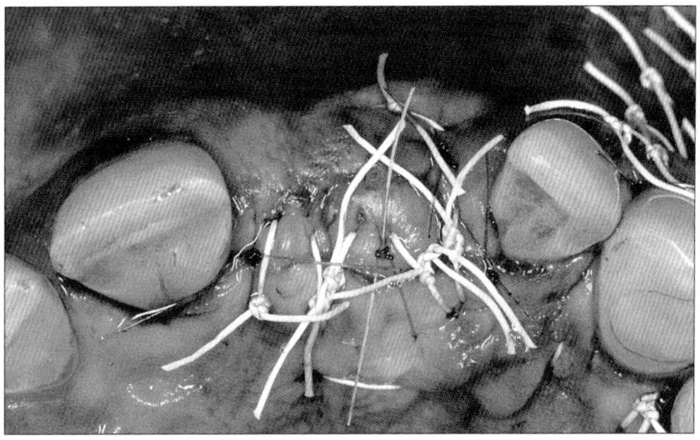

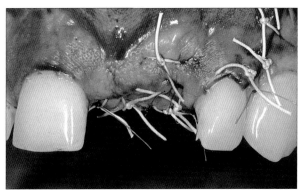

Fig 17a   Thin suturing material ensuring proper adaptation of the tissues.

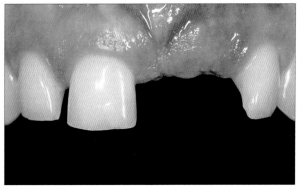

Fig 17b   Thick suturing facilitating safe and stable wound closure.

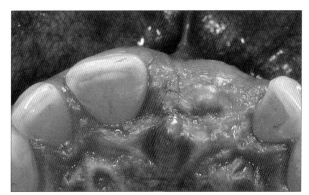

Fig 18a   Healthy soft tissue six months after implantation.

The flap was released via periosteal releasing incisions, and the wound was closed with non-resorbable suturing material. This hydrophobic, non-resorbable e-PTFE membrane material has an increased risk for wound dehiscence compared to resorbable collagen membranes (Zitzmann and coworkers, 1997). In order to ensure proper wound closure, two suturing materials were used, the thicker one for tension and the thinner one for adaptation (Fig 17).

Six months after implant placement, the site was re-evaluated for removal of the membrane (Fig 18a).

The soft tissue was healthy, and a favorable contour of the alveolar arch could be noted (Fig 18b).

Fig 18b   Incisal view of well-healed soft tissue.

After re-entry (Fig 19) and removal of the membrane, the augmentation procedure could be considered a success, as a favorable bone contour and volume were present at the implant site (Fig 20).

The vertical bone height was ideal as bone was present up to the level of the implant shoulder (Fig 20b).

To increase the thickness of the peri-implant mucosa, a connective-tissue graft was harvested from the palate at the time of membrane removal (Fig 21). The graft was sutured to the palatal mucosa and placed over the implant (Fig 22).

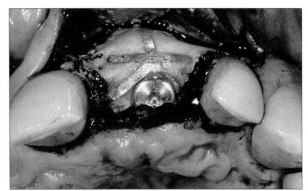

Fig 19   Healing cap facilitating access to the implant shoulder as well as removal of the membrane.

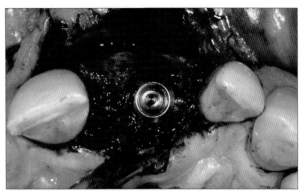

Fig 20a   Augmentation site after membrane removal, showing favorable horizontal bone volume.

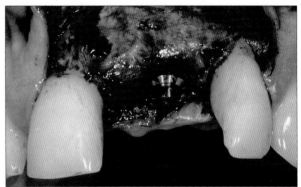

Fig 20b   Favorable vertical bone height after membrane removal.

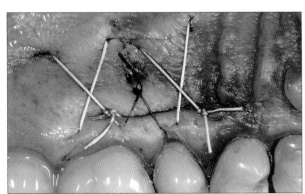

Fig 21   Connective-tissue graft donor site after harvesting and suturing.

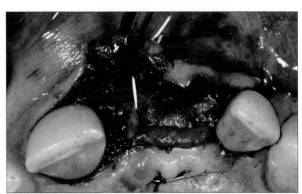

Fig 22   Graft placed over the implant underneath the buccal flap.

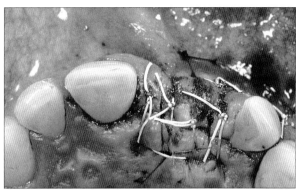

Fig 23   Primary soft-tissue closure with horizontal mattress sutures and single interrupted sutures.

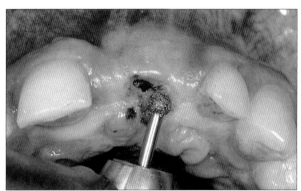

Fig 24   De-epithelialization of the future flap area.

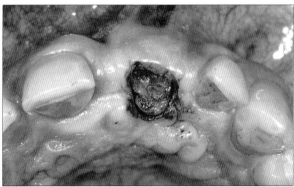

Fig 25   Flap creation above the implant.

Primary soft-tissue closure was again achieved (Fig 23).

Six weeks after soft-tissue augmentation, the reopening procedure for the insertion of a healing cap was initiated. To increase root prominence at the prospective implant site, a small-pedicle rotation flap was created above the implant.

The area was de-epithelialized with a high-speed angled handpiece and a ball-shaped diamond bur (Fig 24).

After de-epithelialization, a U-shaped incision was made above the implant shoulder, with the opening of the U pointing toward the labial aspect (Fig 25).

This pedicled flap was mobilized and positioned between the implant neck and the labial mucosa (Figs 26, 27).

After this procedure, a labially beveled healing cap was inserted onto the implant to ensure access to the implant shoulder and to start the soft-tissue conditioning phase (Fig 28).

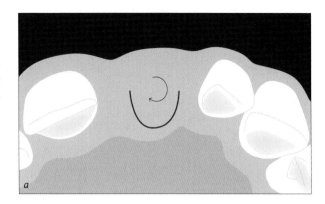

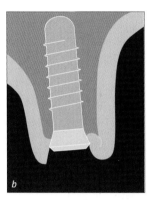

Figs 26a, b   Labially pedicled flap, carefully tucked under in a labial direction.

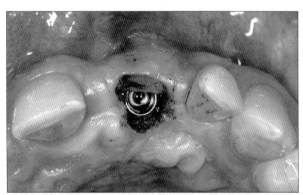

Fig 27   Rotated flap improving the labial contour of the implant site.

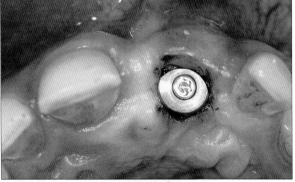

Fig 28   Healing cap helping stabilize the flap.

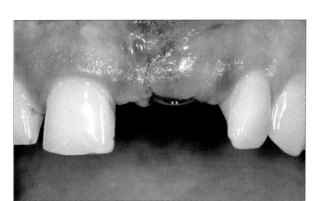

Fig 29   Favorable soft tissue height and volume.

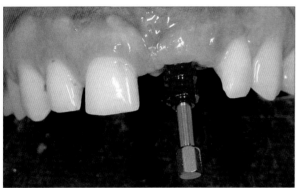

Fig 30   Impression cap screwed to the implant.

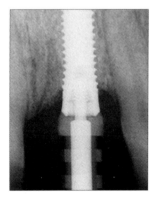

Fig 31   Precise seating of the impression cap on the implant shoulder ensures a precise impression.

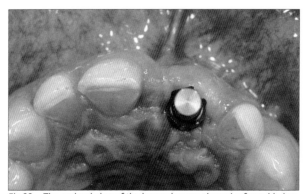

Fig 32   The occlusal view of the impression cap showed a favorable buccooral implant position for the screw-retained superstructure.

The pedicle rotation flap helps increase soft-tissue thickness, creating a favorable contour.

The situation from the labial aspect after the preparation of the pedicle rotation flap and the insertion of the healing cap is shown in Figure 29.

Two weeks later, a screw-retained impression cap was inserted onto the implant for impression-taking and the subsequent fabrication of a temporary crown (Fig 30).

The periapical radiograph showed that the cap was correctly seated on the implant shoulder without forming any marginal gaps (Fig 31).

The radiograph also showed that the implant was successfully placed in the planned position. Furthermore, the implant was well osseointegrated.

The implant axis allows the fabrication of a transocclusally screw-retained superstructure, as evidenced by the position of the impression cap (Fig 32).

A customized impression tray was perforated to allow for loosening the screw of the impression cap after taking the impression. The correct position of the perforation was checked in the patient's mouth (Fig 33).

To ensure easy loosening of the screw and subsequent removal of the impression, the area around the screw was also blocked out with wax (Fig 34).

The impression was sent to the dental lab for fabrication of a cast model. Before pouring the impression, an implant analog was screwed on top of the impression cap (Fig 35).

In the dental lab, the transocclusally screw-retained provisional crown was fabricated on a titanium post for temporary restorations (Fig 36).

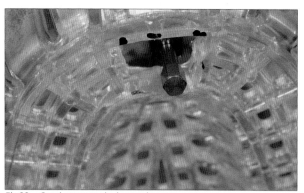

Fig 33   Good access to the impression cap.

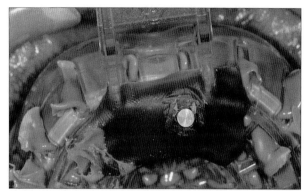

Fig 34   Wax facilitating the loosening of the screw before the impression is removed.

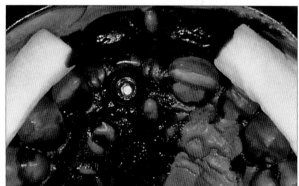

Fig 35   Impression ready for transfer to the dental lab.

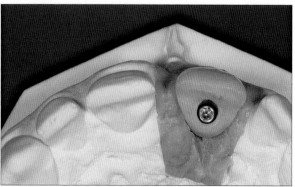

Fig 36   The transocclusally screw-retained provisional crown on the model.

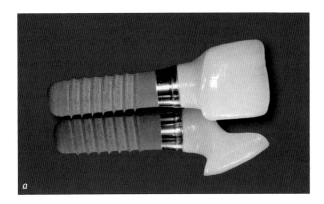

Fig 37   Provisional crown integrating well into the line of natural teeth.

The patient's wish for the diastemas to be retained was met (Fig 37).

The cervical portion of the temporary crown was kept slim on its labial aspect to create the ideal cervical shape at chairside (Fig 38).

Five weeks after reopening and after the insertion of the healing cap, the soft tissues were healthy and well-maintained. Note the favorable soft-tissue volume and contours at the implant site (Fig 39).

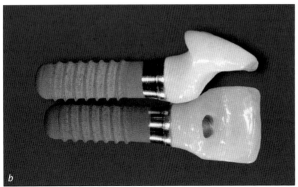

Figs 38a, b   Cervical portion of the crown to be shaped chairside.

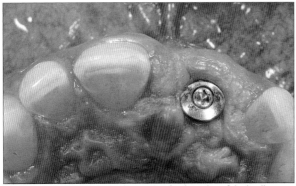

Fig 39   The clinical situation five weeks after insertion of the healing cap.

The labial view showed that special care was needed to create esthetic soft-tissue contours and interdental papillae (Fig 40). The following soft-tissue conditioning procedure helped create a more favorable soft-tissue contour.

After the healing cap was removed, the mucosa was stable and well established (Fig 41).

To condition the peri-implant mucosa to the desired emergence profile and contour, the cervical portion of the provisional crown was modified accordingly, applying a flowable light-curing composite material in a chairside procedure (Fig 42).

The application of the composite material was driven by the point of emergence of the crown. The goal was to copy and match the line of the marginal gingiva at contralateral tooth 11.

At insertion of the provisional crown, notable blanching of the mucosa occurred (Fig 43).

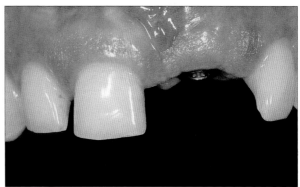

Fig 40   A flat mucosal contour at the implant site.

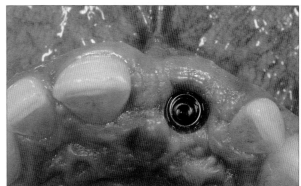

Fig 41   After removal of the healing cap.

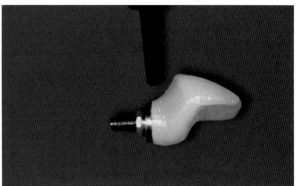

Fig 42   Stepwise adaptation of the cervical portion of the provisional.

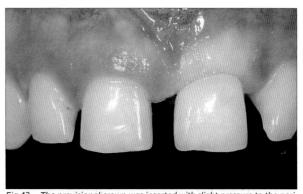

Fig 43   The provisional crown was inserted with slight pressure to the peri-implant mucosa.

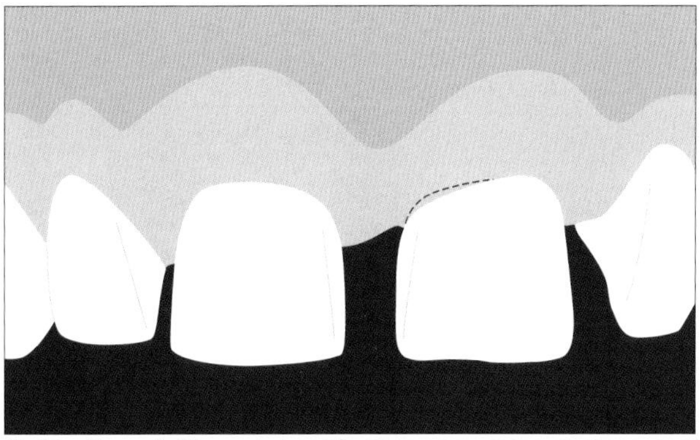

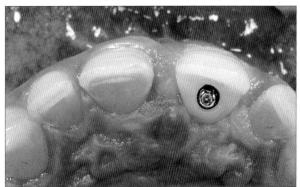

Fig 44   The goal of the cervical modification process was to make the course of the mucosa match the course of the gingiva at tooth 11 as closely as possible. This was achieved by adding composite material in the respective areas.

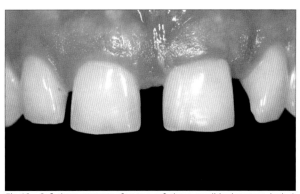

Fig 45   The provisional crown from the incisal aspect.

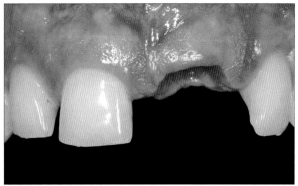

Fig 46   Soft-tissue contour after two soft-tissue conditioning steps, including modification of the provisional crown.

Step by step, composite material was added where the mucosa line needed to be improved (Fig 44).

The pressure applied to the mucosa by the cervical portion of the temporary crown allowed the desired emergence profile. Due to the ideal implant axis, the provisional crown could be transocclusally screw-retained (Fig 45).

After two to four weeks, additional soft-tissue conditioning can take place to further improve the emergence profile and the line of the marginal mucosa.

Another two to four weeks later, a final soft-tissue conditioning step can be made if necessary. In this case, a pleasing soft-tissue contour was found after two soft-tissue conditioning steps (Fig 46).

Also, a favorable increase in soft-tissue height between the two central incisors was seen.

Soft-tissue maturation takes place during the first three to six months after reopening and the insertion of the healing cap and the provisional, respectively. During this time, buccal soft-tissue recession may be expected (Grunder, 2000).

To prevent recession after the insertion of the final crown, the provisional crown is kept in place for at least 3 to 6 months in general (Fig 47).

Fig 47   Clinical situation at the end of the soft-tissue conditioning phase, labial view.

This final soft-tissue shape had to be transferred to the dental lab as precisely as possible (Fig 48).

To capture this final tissue shape, an individual impression cap was fabricated by placing the provisional on an implant analog (Fig 49) and pressing it into silicone.

The individual impression cap was then attached to the implant in the patient's mouth with the integral screw (Fig 50).

The individualized impression cap prevented the soft tissues from collapsing and ensured precise modeling of the emergence profile for the fabrication of the final crown (Fig 51).

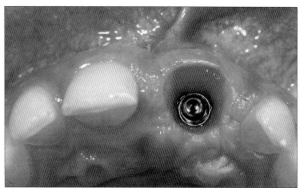

Fig 48   Clinical situation at the end of the soft-tissue conditioning phase, incisal view.

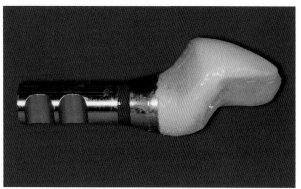

Fig 49   The shape of the provisional crown to be transferred to the impression cap.

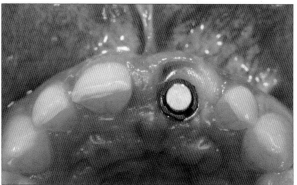

Fig 50   Individualized impression cap perfectly supporting the mucosa.

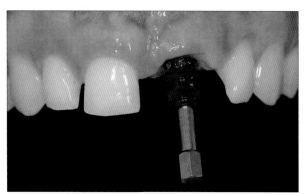

Fig 51   Well-supported labial aspect of the mucosa.

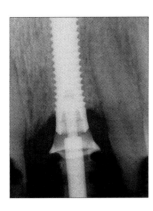

Fig 52   Individualized impression cap seated on the implant shoulder without marginal gaps.

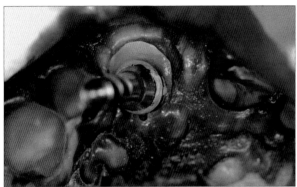

Fig 53   Impression being prepared for fabricating the cast.

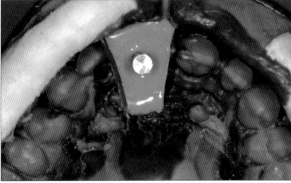

Fig 54   The fabrication of a gingiva mask is recommended in esthetic sites.

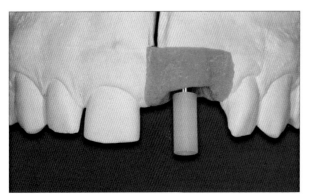

Fig 55   The synOcta gold coping attached to the implant analog.

The precise seating of the impression cap on the implant shoulder was radiologically checked one more time (Fig 52).

In the dental laboratory, an implant analog was attached to the individual impression cap for master cast fabrication (Fig 53).

Silicone material was applied to the implant site to create a gingiva mask (Fig 54).

After the fabrication of the final master cast, a decision must be made concerning the abutment type selection. Due to the scalloped gingival line, cementation at the level of the implant shoulder is not recommended because of the difficult access for cement removal, especially in the interdental area. Cementation of an individual abutment or a screw-retained reconstruction should be chosen. The favorable implant position allowed a screw-retained reconstruction in this particular case.

A Regular-Neck (RN) synOcta gold coping was screwed onto the implant analog for fabrication of a transocclusally screw-retained ceramo-metal crown (Fig 55).

The metal core of the future crown was modeled in wax (Fig 56). A silicone key representing the diagnostic waxup was used to determine the ideal shape and dimension of the metal core.

Figure 57 shows the crown's cast-metal frame.

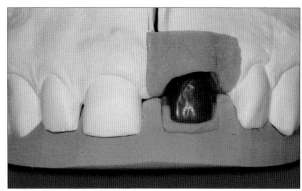

Fig 56a   The waxup, labial view.

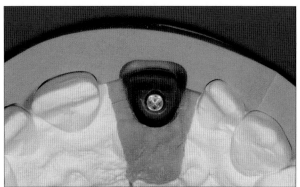

Fig 56b   The waxup, incisal view.

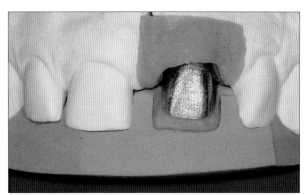

Fig 57a   The cast-metal crown framework, labial view.

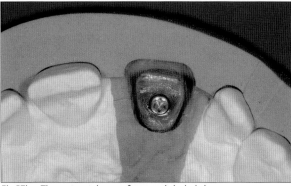

Fig 57b   The cast-metal crown framework, incisal view.

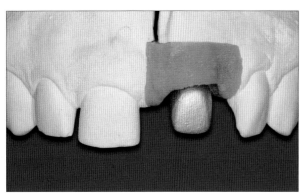

Fig 58   Gold bonder applied, labial view with gingiva mask.

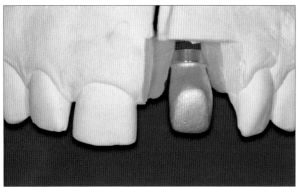

Fig 59   Gold bonder applied, labial view without gingiva mask.

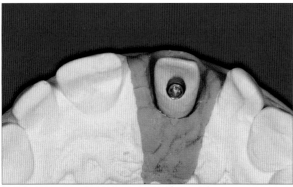

Fig 60   Opaque applied to the cast-metal framework.

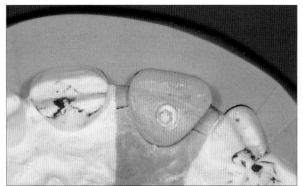

Fig 61   Occlusion check on the model.

After preparing the gold framework with corundum stones at low speed, the framework was cleaned in ethanol for 10 minutes. Gold bonder was evenly applied and baked on in order to shift the color from "cold gray" to "warm gold" (Figs 58, 59).

Opaque was applied (Fig 60), and the veneering ceramic was built up using the layering technique.

Again, a silicone key was used to determine the ideal shape of the crown (Fig 61).

The occlusion was carefully checked, and disturbances were removed in order to establish anterior tooth guidance (Fig 61).

Figures 62 and 63 show the crown as it was ready for insertion (Figs 62, 63).

The final crown integrated very well with the natural dentition with regard to tooth shape, size, color, and surface texture. The line of the incisal edges and the line of the gingival and mucosal margins were harmonious and contributed to the esthetically pleasing treatment outcome (Fig 64).

The treatment was in line with the patient's wishes and could be considered an esthetic success (Fig 65).

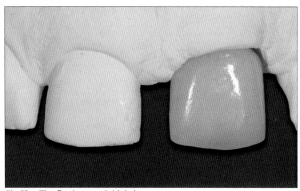

Fig 62   The final crown, labial view.

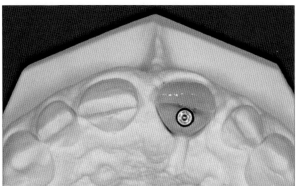

Fig 63   The final crown, incisal view.

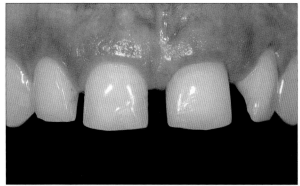

Fig 64   The implant-supported superstructure in situ.

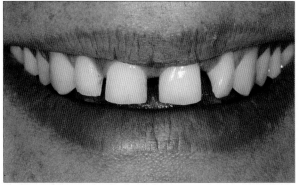

Fig 65   At full natural smile, the implant-supported crown cannot be distinguished from the natural teeth.

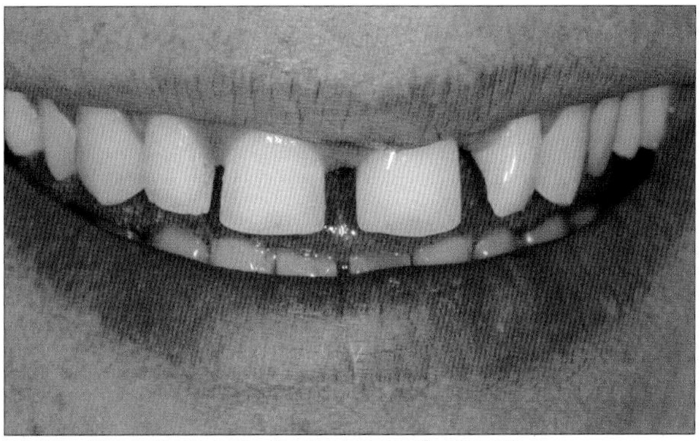

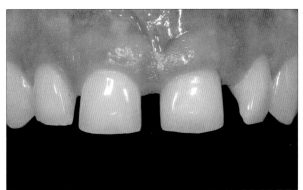

Fig 66   The patient's smile line thee years after insertion.

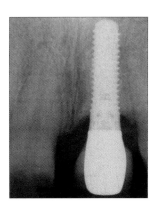

Fig 67   Healthy peri-implant soft tissue and a stable esthetic treatment outcome.

Fig 68   Periapical radiograph three years after implant insertion.

At the patient's follow-up visit three years later, the esthetic treatment outcome was stable (Figs 66 – 68).

Acknowledgments

Prosthetic Procedures
Contribution to the surgical procedure by Dr. Vincent Goh – University of Zurich, Switzerland, Clinic for Dental Crown and Bridge Prosthetics, Partial Prosthetics, and Dental Material Science

Laboratory Procedures
Dental Technician Daniel Pally – University of Zurich, Switzerland, Clinic for Dental Crown and Bridge Prosthetics, Partial Prosthetics, and Dental Material Science

Replacement of an Upper Left Central Incisor with a Regular Neck Implant, Restored with a Ceramo-Metal Crown, Transocclusally Screw-Retained

U. C. Belser

In September 2004, a 38-year-old female patient, a non-smoker, was referred to our clinic for the replacement of the missing left central maxillary incisor (tooth 21), which had been removed two months before the initial appointment due to a vertical root fracture. The dental patient history revealed that the tooth in question had supported a ceramo-metal crown for more than ten years before the root fracture occurred.

Implant therapy (single-tooth replacement) was considered the first therapeutic choice, as the neighboring teeth did not require significant restoration.

The patient was in good general health, and her medical history revealed no significant findings.

At full smile, the patient presented a high lip-line situation, displaying full teeth and associated gingival tissue in the anterior maxilla (Fig 1). The patient's gingival biotype was thin to medium thick and highly scalloped, associated with a broad band of keratinized mucosa.

The initial intraoral radiograph displayed the characteristic status to be expected after the recent extraction of a root (in this particular case of tooth 21). The outline of the alveolus was still clearly visible. Furthermore, the radiograph confirmed the presence of sufficient intact interproximal bone at both adjacent teeth (Fig 2).

Clinical examination of the anterior maxilla revealed the presence of a harmoniously scalloped soft-tissue line and the absence of significant vertical-tissue loss (Fig 3). Together with the relevant radiographic findings, this indicated that the initial clinical situation greatly favored implant therapy for single-tooth replacement.

The above findings led to the following patient-specific esthetic risk profile (Table 1), which could be classified as medium.

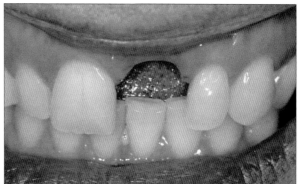

Fig 1   At full smile, the high lip line showed a significant portion of the gingival tissue.

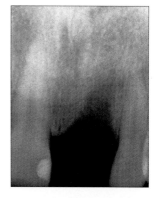

Fig 2   Initial intraoral radiograph showing both the typical situation after a recent tooth extraction (tooth 21) and the presence of intact interproximal bone tissue with sufficient height at the two adjacent roots.

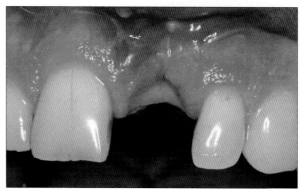

Fig 3   The labial close-up view of the anterior maxilla demonstrated a basically unaltered line of the vestibular soft tissue line with intact interproximal tissue of sufficient height at the two natural teeth adjacent to the extraction site.

Table 1   *The patient's individual esthetic risk profile.*

Esthetic Risk Factors	Low	Medium	High
Medical status	Healthy and cooperative patient with intact immune system		Reduced immune system
Smoking habit	Non-smoker	Light smoker (≤ 10 cig/d)	Heavy smoker (> 10 cig/d)
Patient's esthetic expectations	Low	Medium	High
Lip line	Low	Medium	High
Gingival biotype	Low scalloped, thick	Medium scalloped, medium thick	High scalloped, thin
Shape of tooth crowns	Rectangular		Triangular
Infection at implant site	None	Chronic	Acute
Bone level at adjacent teeth	≤ 5 mm to contact point	5.5 to 6.5 mm to contact point	≥ 7 mm to contact point
Restorative status of neighboring teeth	11: minimally restored 22: virgin		Restored
Width of edentulous span	1 tooth (≥ 7 mm)	1 tooth (< 7 mm)	2 teeth or more
Soft-tissue anatomy	Intact soft tissue		Soft-tissue defects
Bone anatomy of alveolar crest	Alveolar crest without bone deficiency	Horizontal bone deficiency	Vertical bone deficiency

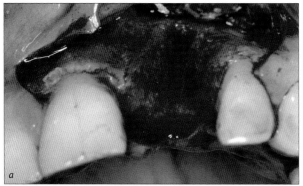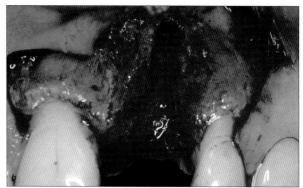

Figs 4a, b   At the moment of flap elevation, i.e. approximately two months after the extraction of the longitudinally fractured root, the prospective implant site 21 presented a localized, bone defect. The degree of horizontal tissue loss could be assessed in a more occlusal view (a), whereas the amount of vertical bone loss became clearly evident on the labial view (b).

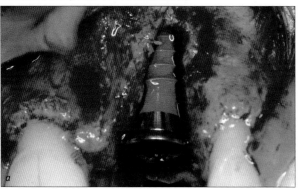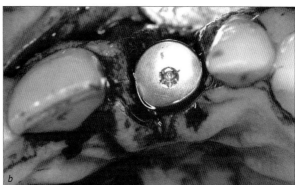

Figs 5a, b   The labial view, immediately after the placement of a standard screw-type implant (a), confirmed the resulting two-wall dehiscence-type defect. The occlusal view clearly documented that the implant had been placed completely inside the alveolar bone crest (b).

The overall complexity of the case corresponded to the advanced level and was associated with a medium esthetic risk. Implant therapy, however, was clearly the number-one choice, as the restorative status of the neighboring teeth did not require full-coverage therapy and because all of the key conditions for the predictable success of single-tooth implant therapy, including the esthetic parameters, were present (Belser and coworkers, 2003; Belser and coworkers, 2004; Buser and coworkers, 2004; Higginbottom and coworkers, 2004).

After elevation of a mucoperiosteal flap, a localized, confined bone defect comprising both a horizontal and a significant vertical component became apparent at site 21 (Figs 4a, b). Despite the obvious hard-tissue defect, this local anatomical situation was considered compatible with the insertion of an implant. This judgment was based on the following elements: the local bone anatomy would permit (1) optimal three-dimensional implant positioning; (2) adequate primary implant stability; and (3) execution of a predictable simultaneous guided bone-regeneration (GBR) procedure.

A standard implant was inserted according to the guidelines described in Chapter 4.1 of this Treatment Guide and achieved adequate primary stability. Furthermore, the entire circumference of the implant could be placed inside the confinement of the surrounding alveolar bone crest, resulting in a three-wall dehiscence-type bony defect that represented conditions favoring a predictable simultaneous GBR procedure (Buser and coworkers, 2004) (Figs 5a, b).

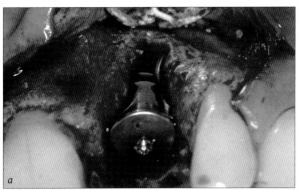 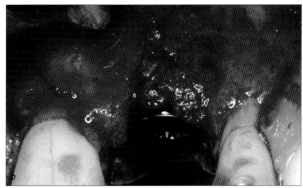

Figs 6a, b   Comparative view of the vestibular aspect of the freshly inserted implant before (a) and after (b) adaptation of small autogenous bone chips collected in the close environment.

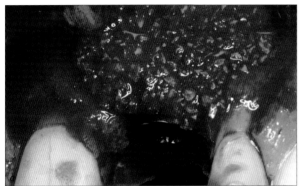 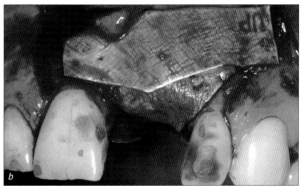

Figs 7a, b   The second step of the simultaneous GBR procedure was the application of a considerable amount of bone fillers (a) in order to recreate in slight excess the originally convex labial contour of the alveolar ridge. To favor the selective in-growth of bone-forming cells, a bio-absorbable barrier membrane was applied in two layers (b), in what is termed "double layer technique."

The resulting vestibular dehiscence-type defect (Fig 6a) was covered with small autogenous bone grafts harvested in the immediate neighborhood of the implant site (Fig 6b).

The next step was to apply a layer of bone fillers soaked with blood (Fig 7a) to rebuild a slightly excessive convex labial contour of the alveolar bone crest. The bone fillers were covered with two layers of a bioabsorbable barrier membrane (Fig 7b) in order to permit the bone-forming cells to invade the wound selectively and ultimately to cover the bone-filler particles with newly formed bone.

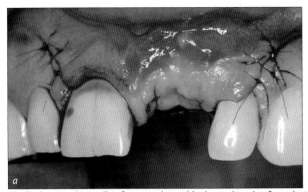 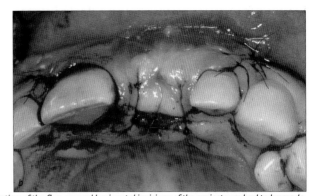

Figs 8a, b   In order to allow for coronal repositioning and tension-free adaptation of the flap, several horizontal incisions of the periosteum had to be made. The occlusal view (b) confirmed the establishment of a labial convexity of the alveolar ridge at the site of implant placement, similar to that observed at the adjacent natural dentition.

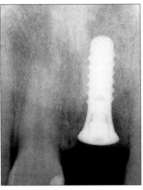

Fig 9   The intraoral radiograph, taken immediately after the insertion of the 12 mm screw-type implant, confirmed an adequate implant position with respect to depth, axis in the frontal plane, and distance toward the adjacent natural roots.

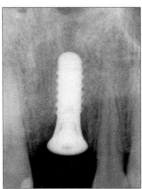

Fig 10   The control radiograph, taken ten weeks after implant placement, showing the extent of initial interproximal peri-implant bone remodeling and the maintenance of the original vertical bone height at the two adjacent natural roots.

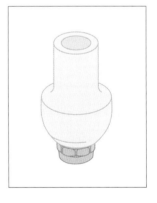

Fig 11   The temporary mesoabutment was used as base for a chairside fabricated screw-retained provisional implant restoration to initiate peri-implant soft-tissue conditioning.

The last step in this combined implant placement/bone augmentation procedure was the precise adaptation of the flap (Figs 8a, b). As a considerable ridge volume had been added in the form of autogenous bone grafts and bone fillers, several horizontal incisions of the periosteum at the base of the flap were required to achieve an accurate and tension-free repositioning of the flap, stabilized by interrupted sutures. The authors consider primary wound closure an integral part of the preferred protocol for the anterior maxilla, in the interest of predictability.

Before dismissing the patient, an intraoral radiograph (Fig 9) was taken to verify the correct implant position with respect to depth, axis, and relation to the neighboring roots and to create a baseline document for future comparison (Fig 10).

In accordance with the recommended early implant placement/early implant restoration concept, the successful osseointegration was verified ten weeks after implant placement, first radiographically (Fig 10) and then clinically.

When it comes to single-tooth replacement in the anterior maxilla, it is generally recommended to use either an implant-borne fixed temporary restoration (usually screw-retained, as the implant shoulder is normally located distinctly submucosally in the interproximal area and thus not easily amenable to cementing), or to utilize a simple "tissue former" component to initiate peri-implant soft-tissue conditioning. The prefabricated Regular Neck (RN) synOcta temporary mesoabutment (Fig 11) serves both these purposes (Priest, 2003; Small and Tarnow, 2000; Giannopoulou and coworkers, 2004; Jemt, 1999).

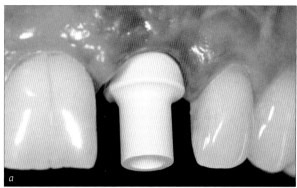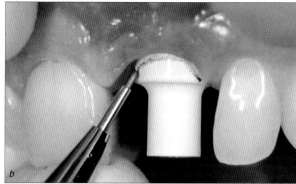

Figs 12a, b   Having reduced the cervical emergence profile of the prefabricated temporary component on its interproximal and labial aspects, the meso-abutment was connected directly to the implant with the integrated occlusal screw (a). The precise level and course of the marginal soft-tissue line was marked with a pencil (b).

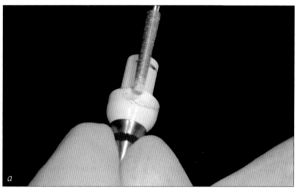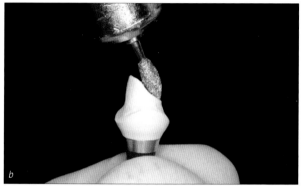

Figs 13a, b   Necessary individual modifications were performed outside the oral cavity wherever possible, using the appropriate rotary instruments. For that purpose, the mesoabutment was attached to a laboratory analog with its integrated occlusal screw.

The respective prosthetic component was connected directly to the implant shoulder via its integrated occlusal screw (Fig 12a), after first verifying and eventually correcting the cervical emergence profile, which may be too "bulky" in a given clinical situation. It is important not to compress the mucosa excessively, particularly in its vestibular aspect, as this may lead to soft-tissue recession with negative consequences for esthetic appearance. The next step was to circumferentially mark the level and course of the peri-implant mucosal margin (Fig 12b).

The marked mesoabutment was attached to the corresponding RN laboratory analog to facilitate the necessary modifications, which were performed with appropriate diamond burs and abrasive disks (Figs 13a, b). To increase the efficacy (precision and time) of the procedure and to minimize potential sources of tissue irritation, all the corrections that could be carried out outside the oral cavity were made on the implant analog.

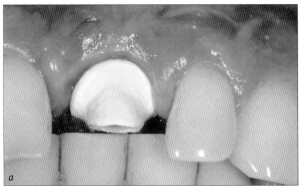 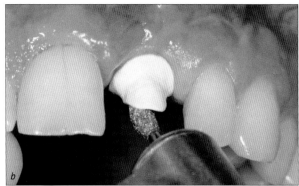

Figs 14a, b   The customized temporary mesoabutment was reattached to the implant, secured with its retention screw, and the occlusal features carefully verified (a) and then corrected intraorally using diamond burs (b).

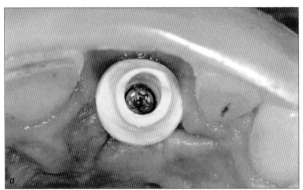 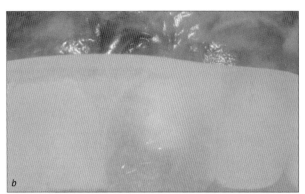

Figs 15a, b   A transparent silicone material was used to verify the space at disposition for the subsequent acrylic resin veneering of the customized temporary mesoabutment. This newly developed type of material is characterized by its high level of precision and the additional possibility to use light-curing acrylic resins, which in turn was significantly contributing to the efficacy of the described chair-side procedure.

Before completing the temporary component with acrylic resin, an intraoral try-in was performed to verify that the adjustments corresponded to the individual clinical needs (Figs 14a, b). In particular, the occlusal requirements were minutely verified and further corrections carried out directly in the patient's mouth where indicated.

A transparent silicone key helped precisely assess the space available for the acrylic resin to be used for veneering (Figs 15a, b). The recent introduction of transparent silicone materials made it possible to use intraoral high-precision templates for direct provisional restorations and gave access to light-curing resins. The latter aspect contributes significantly to efficacy in a chairside setting, where time is of paramount importance.

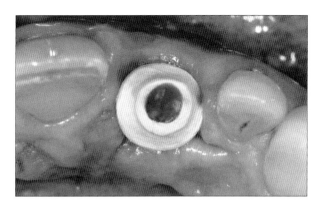

Fig 16   Before proceeding to the intraoral application of light-curing acrylic resin, the screw-access channel was blocked out with wax to guarantee easy and rapid access to the occlusal screw immediately after polymerization of the light-curing material directly in the patient's mouth.

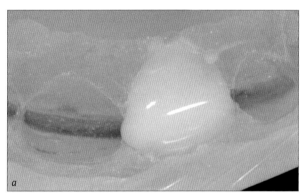

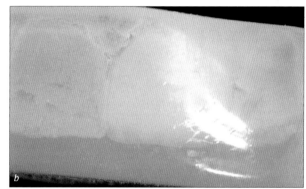

Figs 17a, b   An advantage of using a combination of a transparent silicone material and a light-polymerizing acrylic resin is that the key can be carefully loaded, the absence of air entrapments can be verified, and the subsequent intraoral positioning carried out without time constraints. The light-curing process itself is extremely rapid and has no clinical shortcomings such as tissue irritation caused by free monomers and an increase in temperature.

A direct (chairside) screw-retained provisional implant restoration had been planned for this patient. The respective screw-access channel was blocked out with wax before the acrylic resin was applied (Fig 16) to assure easy access to the screw once the acrylic resin was processed – a simple measure taken to render this chairside procedure as safe and as fast as possible for the benefit of both the patient and the clinician.

Another advantage of using a combination of a transparent silicone key and a light-curing acrylic resin is that they provide abundant time for careful loading of the silicone template at the corresponding location and for verifying the absence of any air entrapments (Figs 17a, b). Once this check had been made and any "bubbles" had been eliminated, the key was precisely repositioned on the dental arch, followed by a short time of exposure to the curing light. The template was removed, the access to the screw-access channel was established, and the restoration was removed from the patient's mouth, attached to the laboratory analog, and all correction and finishing procedures were performed extraorally.

Figs 18a, b   The lateral close-up view of the finalized provisional implant restoration before and after its insertion, showing that a flat cervical emergence profile was established. Note the smooth transition from the prefabricated temporary mesoabutment to the secondary acrylic resin (a). Immediately after insertion of the provisional in the patient's mouth (b), only minimal blanching of the peri-implant soft tissue occurred, and an acceptable overall esthetic integration of the provisional was observed.

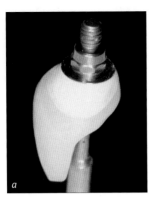
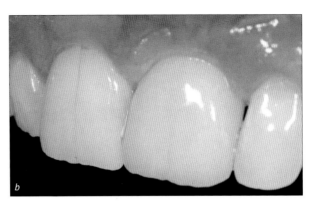

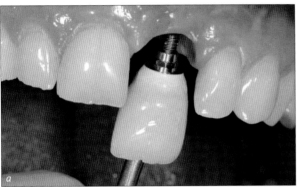
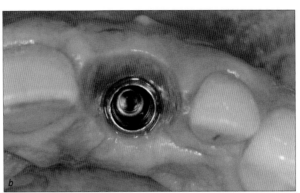

Figs 19a, b   Two months after insertion of the screw-retained implant provisional, the peri-implant soft tissue displayed healthy and stable features. From an esthetic point of view, the soft-tissue appearance and contours were favorable. At this stage, the clinical situation was judged adequate for taking the final impression.

After the completion phase of the temporary implant restoration, which comprises its general shape, cervical emergence profile, interproximal contacts, occlusal features, surface texture characteristics, and shade, the provisional can be either mechanically polished or glazed with a light-curing varnish and subsequently inserted in the patient's mouth (Figs 18a, b). This step in the chain of reconstructive procedures initiated the phase of peri-implant soft-tissue conditioning to create a healthy, stable, and esthetic mucosal configuration.

Approximately two months after the placement of the implant provisional, the peri-implant soft-tissue configuration was considered adequate for undertaking the next treatment step, consisting of final impression taking. A carefully fabricated implant provisional, as previously described, in conjunction with a well-instructed and highly compliant patient as far as plaque control and maintenance were concerned, led to optimal peri-implant soft-tissue conditions, including esthetic mucosal contours (Figs 19a, b).

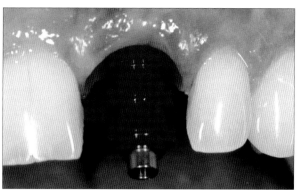

Fig 20   In the presence of a distinctly submucosal implant shoulder, an open-tray type impression was performed using a screw-retained impression cap. Care was taken to proceed with impression-taking immediately after removing the provisional in order to pick up a maximum amount of the relevant peri-implant soft-tissue contours created by the axial profile of the temporary restoration.

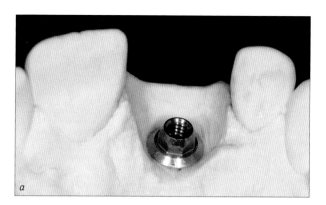

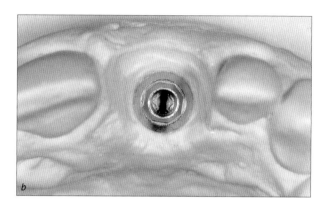

One of the major reasons for fabricating a provisional implant restoration had been to generate stable and esthetic peri-implant soft-tissue contours, similar to those observed at the natural control tooth. At the same time, the patient's compliance concerning oral hygiene, which can be particularly demanding when it comes to an implant restoration in the esthetic zone, could be monitored and reinforced if necessary. The patient's capacity to use e.g. Superfloss daily and efficiently had an impact on the design of the final restoration, especially in regard to its axial profile. It is well known that this can be "more hygienic, but less esthetic" or vice versa.

In this particular patient, compliance was considered optimal and the resulting soft-tissue conditions were fully compatible with a highly esthetic superstructure design. Two impressions of the maxilla were taken: (1) an alginate impression with the temporary still in place (to guide the laboratory technician during the fabrication of the final implant-supported crown), and (2) a final elastomeric impression to produce the master cast. As in most instances in the anterior maxilla, an open-tray impression in association with a screw-retained impression cap was chosen, primarily because the implant shoulder was located distinctly submucosally (Fig 20).

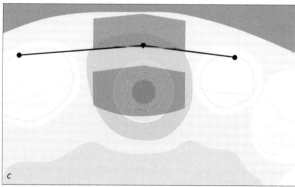

Figs 21a-c   Close-up views (a: palatal; b: occlusal) of the master cast documenting the optimal implant position in an orofacial and a mesiodistal direction. The implant was ideally placed within the orofacial and mesiodistal comfort zones (c).

Care was taken to proceed with impression-taking immediately after removing the provisional, in order to pick up a maximum amount of the relevant peri-implant soft-tissue contours created by the axial profile of the temporary restoration. This aspect has clinical significance, as the respective soft tissue tends to collapse rapidly in the direction of the surface of the impression cap and to no longer correspond to the provisional-derived contours. Where this aspect is of major concern, the technique of customizing the impression cap, using the pertinent information derived from the cervical part of the successful temporary restoration, can be applied (as described in Chapter 4.2 of this Treatment Guide).

In most instances, dental technicians, and particularly experienced ceramists, recommend the fabrication of a straightforward stone master cast comprising the integrated laboratory implant analog(s), as in this case (Figs 21a, b). In order to assure adequate access to the shoulder of the implant analog and to create optimal technical conditions for developing an adequate emergence profile of the ceramo-metal restoration, the peri-implant soft tissue was reshaped using rotary instruments. This procedure was based on the information provided by the circumferential line of emergence of the contralateral natural tooth that served as reference. Together with the study cast, representing the provisional implant restoration that had functioned successfully in the patient's mouth for two months, these landmarks represented the basis for the final implant-supported crown.

In this case, the RN synOcta gold coping, a prefabricated restorative implant component permitting a cast-on laboratory procedure, was used to generate the metal framework for the planned transocclusally screw-retained ceramo-metal superstructure.

Using the silicone key derived from the provisional, the ceramist subsequently proceeded with the mounting of the various layers of different ceramic substrates to achieve an optimal reproduction of shapes and optical properties as present in the natural contralateral tooth. This procedure required an "over-build" of crown volume to anticipate the subsequent sintering contraction (Fig 22a). After the first ceramic firing, the volume contraction was particularly evident at the interproximal surfaces, resulting in an absence of interdental contacts (Fig 22b) and requiring at least one additional correction-sintering step.

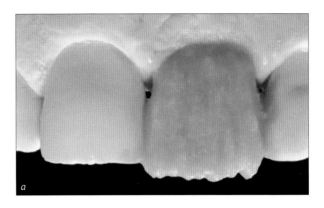

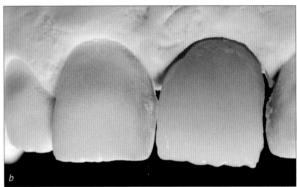

Figs 22a, b In the first step, the clinical crown body was established, composed of a complex sequence of layers of different opacities and shades aimed at imitating the basic components – dentin, enamel, and incisal translucency – of a natural central maxillary incisor (a). After the first ceramic sintering step, a significant volume contraction was observed, requiring at least one additional corrective step. The basic optic tooth-like properties, however, were already clearly visible.

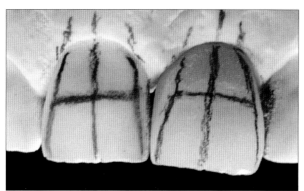

Fig 23   In order to reproduce the main morphological features of the natural control tooth, these elements, such as mesial and distal transition line angles and the long axis of the clinical crown, were first marked on the contralateral tooth and then highlighted on the ceramic crown.

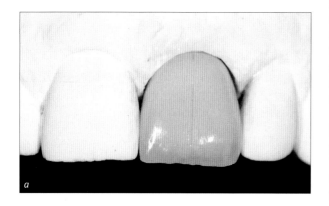

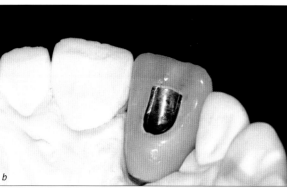

Figs 24a, b   Vestibular and palatal close-up views of the completed transocclusally screw-retained ceramo-metal implant-supported crown.

After the second ceramic firing, the ceramist outlined in pencil the key morphological parameters on both the natural contralateral tooth and on the newly produced ceramo-metal implant-supported crown (Fig 23). This systematic approach ultimately achieved an adequate level of similarity, a determinant for the final esthetic outcome.

After an additional sintering step, the transocclusally screw-retained ceramo-metal implant-supported crown 21 was finalized and mechanically polished to the same characteristic surface texture observed at tooth 11 (Figs 24a, b). For reasons of mechanical strength and to prevent ceramic fractures, the screw-access channel was protected with a metal sleeve.

At the insertion of the final ceramo-metal implant-supported crown, the peri-implant soft tissue presented itself as healthy, stable, and esthetic in appearance (Figs 25a-d). This included the symmetry of the labial line of the mucosa when comparing the implant site with its natural control tooth 11, as well as the appearance of the soft tissue that was free of any signs of inflammation.

The implant-supported crown was inserted in the nearly optimal clinical environment previously described (Fig 26).

As expected under such conditions, the integration of the new implant-supported crown in the adjacent natural dentition reached acceptable standards. A slight vertical soft-tissue loss on both the mesial and distal aspects of the new restoration led to the presence of two small so-called "black triangles." However, this limited degree of soft-tissue loss is still largely within the limits of what one would consider acceptable from an esthetic point of view.

From a radiological point of view, the single-tooth replacement 21 was to be considered successful (Fig 27). The peri-implant bone appeared stable, confirming that osseointegration had reached the steady state, and the interproximal bone height at the two adjacent natural teeth was similar to the preoperative situation.

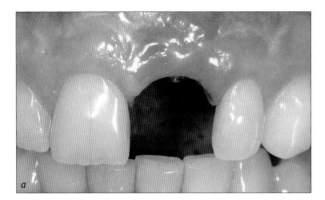
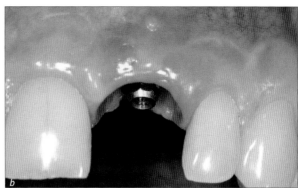

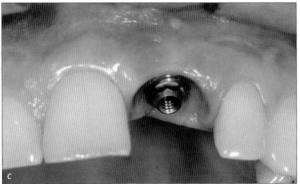
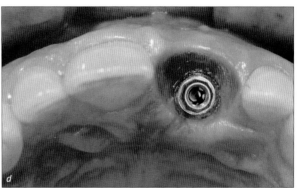

Figs 25a-d Four different close-up views of implant site 21, documenting the almost perfect condition of the peri-implant soft tissue from the points of view of health and esthetics.

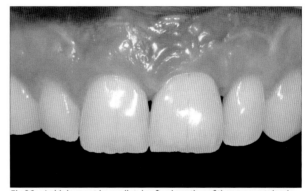

Fig 26 Labial aspect immediately after insertion of the screw-retained ce-ramo-metal implant-supported crown 21, confirming esthetic integration in a natural environment.

Fig 27 Final radiograph confirm-ing a stable peri-implant bone situ-ation, excellent radio-opacity of the precious-alloy substructure, and a good marginal fit of the metal-ce-ramic implant-supported crown.

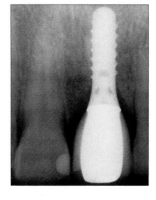

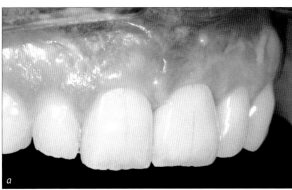 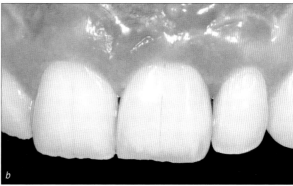

Figs 28a, b   Right and left oblique views, confirming that, despite the slight difference in mesiodistal dimensions between the implant and natural tooth, an esthetically acceptable level of outcome had been reached.

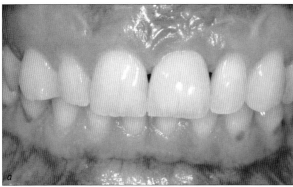 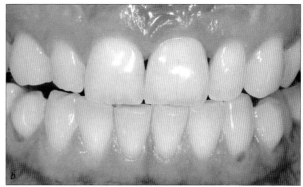

Figs 29a, b   Direct comparison between the centric occlusal position (a) and protrusive excursion of the mandible (b), demonstrating a harmonious occlusal pattern.

When analyzing the esthetic integration from different angles (Figs 28a, b), it became apparent that despite a slight discrepancy between the mesiodistal dimension of the edentulous site 21 and its natural contralateral tooth 11, the basic shapes of the new crown were sufficiently similar to those of its natural model, assuring a largely acceptable outcome.

Functionally, a harmonious anterior guidance, evenly distributing contacts between the two maxillary central incisors during protrusive excursions of the mandible, was established (Fig 29a, b).

At normal communication distance, looking at the patient smiling unforced (Fig 30), an overall acceptable level of integration of the implant-supported single crown was reached from both an esthetic and a functional point of view.

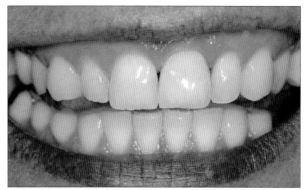

Fig 30   *The patient's unforced smile. Despite a high lip-line situation, an acceptable level of esthetic integration was reached with single-tooth replacement therapy.*

Acknowledgments

Surgical Procedures
Dr. Daniel Buser – Professor, University of Bern, Switzerland, Department of Oral Surgery and Stomatology

Laboratory Procedures
Master Dental Technician Dominique Vinci, University of Geneva, Switzerland

4.10 Replacement of an Upper Right Central Incisor with a Regular Neck Implant Restored with a Ceramo-Metal Crown, Transocclusally Screw-Retained

W.C. Martin

A healthy 32-year-old male patient presented at the clinic for a consultation on treatment options to replace his failing central incisors and retained deciduous canine. This case review addresses the treatment of the central incisors. At full smile, the patient exhibited a medium lip line with tapered clinical crowns and a thin-gingiva biotype (Fig 1).

A retracted view of the central incisors showed a discrepancy in the gingival margin positions of teeth 11 and 21 (Figs 2a-c).

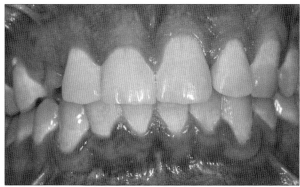

Fig 2a   The retracted view showing clinical crowns with thin scalloped papillae and a moderate band of keratinized tissue.

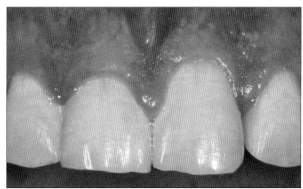

Fig 2b   Frontal view highlighting the discrepancy between the gingival margins of teeth 11 and 21. The gingival margin of tooth 21 is the favorable margin position.

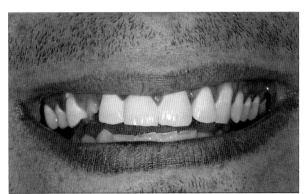

Fig 1   Full smile. Medium lip line exposing the majority of the clinical crowns and the tips of the papillae.

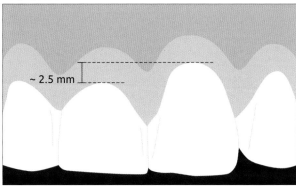

~ 2.5 mm

Fig 2c   The marginal discrepancy between 11 and 21.

A radiographic examination revealed that teeth 11 and 21 were subject to external and internal resorption and that an impacted canine was present (Fig 3). A clinical and radiographic examination showed good circumferential bone support of the anterior teeth. A detailed examination was performed to determine the esthetic risk profile for this patient.

After the consultation, the data obtained were compiled for the esthetic risk-assessment table (Table 1).

Taking into consideration the patient's restorative wishes as well as his medium lip line, thin-gingiva biotype, resorption of the central incisors, and impacted canine, several treatment options were considered. The overall esthetic risk for this treatment is high, indicating that the potential for an esthetic result based upon the ITI Consensus Statements (Belser and coworkers, 2004) for implant restorations is uncertain. The high esthetic risk for this patient is influenced by the need to replace the central incisors. The replacement of the adjacent teeth in the esthetic zone would be a complex process due to the influence of the dental implants on the interimplant bone support. If the possibility of retaining one of the central incisors had existed, the esthetic risk could be adjusted to medium. Based on an understanding of these challenges, alternatives were explored to preserve tooth 21. In addition, the removal of the impacted canine would result in a large osseous defect, so a CT scan was made to help locate the exact position of the impacted tooth relative to the central incisors. Based upon the information gathered from these diagnostic tests, a definitive treatment plan was drawn up, and the esthetic risk in regard to treatment was reviewed with the patient. Three phases of treatment were anticipated:

1. Endodontic – Non-surgical endodontic treatment of tooth 21 to delay or even arrest the internal resorption process.
2. Surgical – Navigated implant surgery, immediate placement of a Regular Neck (RN), Standard Plus (SP) implant at site 11.
3. Restorative – Provisional restoration and subsequent final restoration, focusing on form, function, and esthetics.

Endodontic therapy was performed on tooth 21 (Fig 4). A bi-annual follow-up was initiated to track any changes within the tooth.

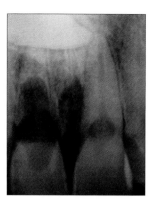

Fig 3   Periapical radiograph showing the advanced internal and external resorption of tooth 11 and moderate internal resorption of tooth 21. The impacted canine is visible, although the extent of the orofacial displacement is not evident.

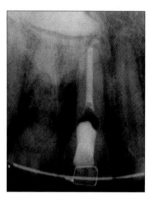

Fig 4   Periapical radiograph after treatment of tooth 21.

Table 1   The patient's individual esthetic risk profile.

Esthetic Risk Factors	Low	Medium	High
Medical status	Healthy and cooperative patient, intact immune system		Reduced immune system
Smoking habit	Non-smoker	Light smoker (≤ 10 cig/d)	Heavy smoker (> 10 cig/d)
Patient's esthetic expectations	Low	Medium	High
Lip line	Low	Medium	High
Gingival biotype	Low-scalloped, thick	Medium scalloped, medium thick	High scalloped, thin
Shape of tooth crowns	Rectangular		Triangular
Infection at implant site	None	Chronic	Acute
Bone level at adjacent teeth	≤ 5 mm to contact point	5.5 to 6.5 mm to contact point	≥ 7 mm to contact point
Restorative status of neighboring teeth	Virgin		Restored
Width of edentulous span	1 tooth (≥ 7 mm)	1 tooth (< 7 mm)	2 teeth or more
Soft-tissue anatomy	Intact soft tissue		Soft-tissue defects
Bone anatomy of alveolar crest	Alveolar crest without bone deficiency	Horizontal bone deficiency	Vertical bone deficiency

Before the surgical session, a custom CT template was fabricated, highlighting the proposed mucosal margin position of tooth 11 (Fig 5).

This template was worn during the CT survey (Fig 6). Information gathered from the survey was analyzed using implant-planning software (DenX Ltd.) In this virtual environment, the dental implant was placed in an ideal position based upon (1) the nature of the planned restoration, (2) available bone, and (3) the position of the impacted canine. At the surgical visit, a periotome was used to remove tooth 11 while maintaining facial bone support.

A navigation system (DenX Ltd.) was used to place a Regular Neck, Standard Plus implant in the ideal three-dimensional position previously planned with the navigation software (Fig 7).

A healing cap was placed and the extracted central incisor was inserted into a vacuform template to be used as an interim restoration. The patient was scheduled for a follow-up visit one week later (Fig 8).

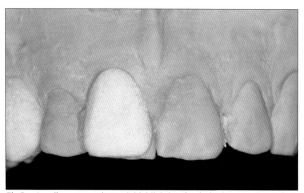

Fig 5   A radiopaque resin tooth highlighting the desired mucosal margin at site 11 was fabricated. This tooth would be incorporated into the CT template.

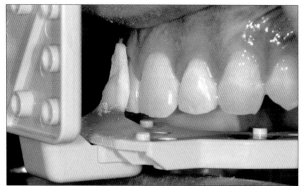

Fig 6   The CT template in place before the radiographic survey.

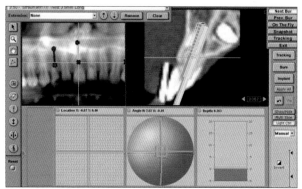

Fig 7   Image of the preparation of the osteotomy during the surgical procedure. The implant was to be placed within the osseous housing and facially of the impacted canine.

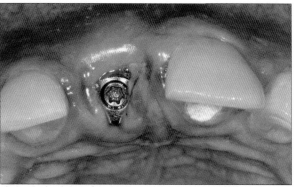

Fig 8   Occlusal view of the healing cap at the one-week follow-up visit.

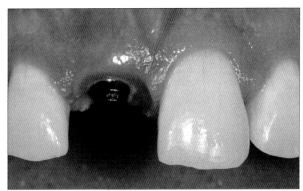

Fig 9   Eight weeks after implant placement.

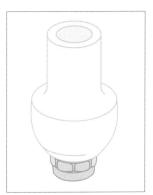

Fig 10   The synOcta temporary mesoabutment.

The patient was scheduled for a loading visit eight weeks after implant placement (Fig 9). At that appointment, a provisional restoration was to be inserted that would initiate the maturation of the transition zone.

Upon removal of the healing cap, excess coronal tissue was evident. A synOcta temporary mesoabutment was selected for use as an interim abutment (Fig 10). A mesoabutment is a prepable peek abutment that allows intraoral modification with a high-speed diamond bur. The key benefits of a mesoabutment are: the placement of a machined connection at the implant shoulder, a preformed emergence profile, and an accessible provisional margin for cement removal.

The abutment was placed on the implant and tightened to 15 Ncm. It was then modified with diamond bur in a high-speed handpiece to create a circumferential submucosal shoulder (Figs 11a, b).

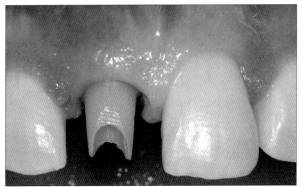

Fig 11a   Frontal view after preparation of the mesoabutment.

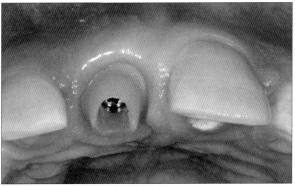

Fig 11b   Occlusal view of the mesoabutment, highlighting the axial position of the implant and circumferential margin preparation.

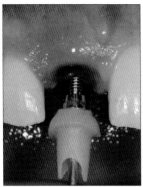 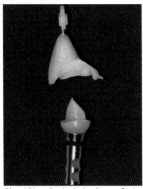 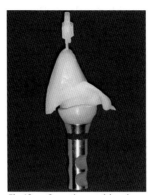 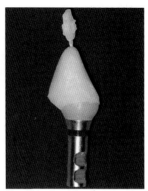

Fig 12a   Frontal view of the meso-abutment during removal.

Fig 12b   Exploded view of the relined polycarbonate crown and mesoabutment on a synOcta analog.

Fig 12c   Once the provisional was placed on the abutment, excess material was removed before building up the ideal emergence profile.

Fig 12d   Provisional restoration and abutment, highlighting the facial and palatal contours.

A prefabricated polycarbonate crown was relined with Triad VLC (Dentsply) over the meso-abutment. The margins of the provisional were refined extraorally to create an ideal emergence contour from the shoulder prepared on the meso-abutment (Figs 12a-d).

Upon completion of the extraoral margination process, the mesoabutment was returned to the mouth and tightened to 15 Ncm. The screw access hole was covered with cotton, and the provisional was cemented with temporary cement (Fig 13). The occlusion was adjusted and the patient scheduled for a final impression after four weeks.

At the return visit, the maturation of the peri-implant tissue could be appreciated (Fig 14).

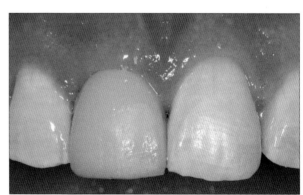

Fig 13   Frontal view after cementation of the provisional restoration.

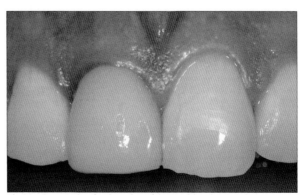

Fig 14   Four weeks after insertion of the provisional restoration.

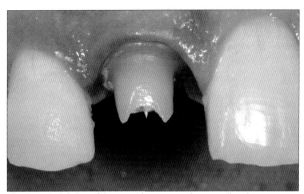

Fig 15a   Facial view of the mesoabutment and surrounding tissue upon removal of the provisional restoration.

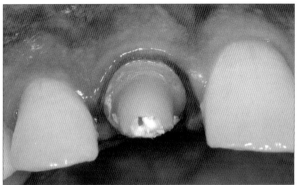

Fig 15b   Occlusal view of the mesoabutment showing minimal inflammation and cement residue.

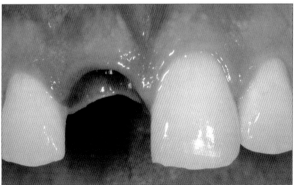

Fig 16a   Facial view of the implant, highlighting the facial and interproximal tissue support.

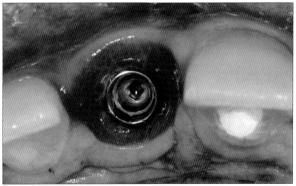

Fig 16b   Occlusal view of the implant and transition zone created by the mesoabutment and provisional restoration.

Upon removal of the provisional restoration, the tissues showed minimal inflammation and little cement residue (Figs 15a-b).

The mesoabutment was removed and the implant cleaned with air and water, allowing the maturation of the transition zone to be appreciated (Figs 16a, b).

Before the final impression, the correct shade was selected (Figs 17a, b).

Due to the large size of the transition zone, a custom impression cap was fabricated at chairside with the aid of the mesoabutment and provisional restoration (Figs 18a-b). The fabrication of a custom impression cap allowed vital information of the transition zone to be transferred to the technician to enhance the final emergence contour of the definitive abutment and restoration.

Upon placement of the customized impression cap, it became evident that full seating could not be confirmed clinically, so a periapical radiograph was taken (Figs 19a, b).

Once full seating had been confirmed, a polyvinyl siloxane impression was made (Fig 20).

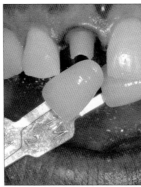 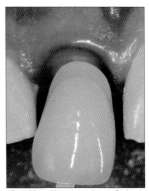

Fig 17a   Shade selection for communication to the laboratory.

Fig 17b   Close-up view of shade tab, highlighting the characterization of the adjacent teeth.

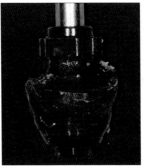 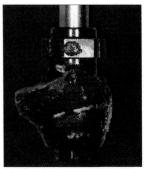

Fig 18a   Frontal view of the custom impression cap, showing the emergence of the transition zone captured with the pattern resin.

Fig 18b   Lateral view of the custom impression cap. The facial emergence profile can be appreciated.

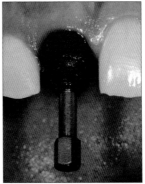 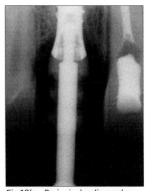

Fig 19a   The frontal view of the custom impression cap in place.

Fig 19b   Periapical radiograph confirming full seating of the custom impression cap.

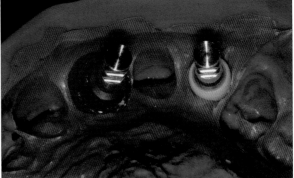

Fig 20   Final impression with the synOcta analogs in place.

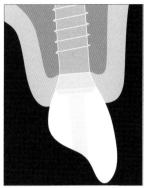

Fig 21   Implant axis passing through the cingulum, allowing for transocclusal screw retention of the crown.

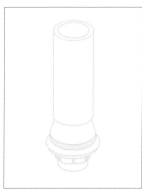

Fig 22   The synOcta gold abutment.

In the laboratory, the position of the implant axis was confirmed as passing through the cingulum of the planned restoration (Fig 21). A screw-retained crown could therefore be selected as the definitive restoration. To accomplish this, a synOcta gold abutment was selected as the definitive abutment (Fig 22). It would allow for the merging of the restoration directly onto the abutment. The result would be a crown that would directly connect into the synOcta connection on the implant, using a single abutment screw to retain the crown on the implant.

The restoration pattern was waxed up to full contour on the master cast, followed by a cut back to allow for the ceramic veneer. After casting, ceramic material was built up and glazed and the fit of the restoration tested on a solid master cast (Figs 23a, b).

The crown and abutment screw were then returned for insertion (Fig 24).

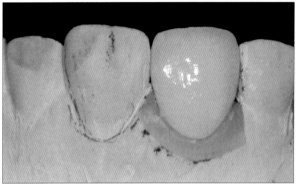

Fig 23a   Final restoration on the master cast.

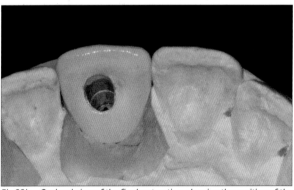

Fig 23b   Occlusal view of the final restoration, showing the position of the screw access hole.

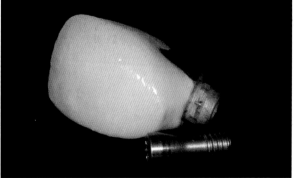

Fig 24   Final crown and abutment screw.

At the insertion visit four weeks after the impression had been taken, the provisional restoration and meso-abutment were removed (Figs 25a, b). The implant was irrigated with an air-water syringe before placing the final crown.

Once the fit and shade of the final restoration had been confirmed, it was tightened to 35 Ncm (Figs 26a, b). The screw access hole was covered with a cotton pellet and sealed with composite. The occlusion was adjusted to a light shimstock pull. Adjustments to the ceramic surface were followed by a polishing procedure with diamond-impregnated disks that helped create a glaze-like ceramic surface.

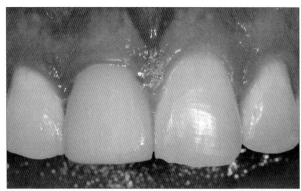

Fig 25a   Frontal view of the provisional restoration at the insertion visit.

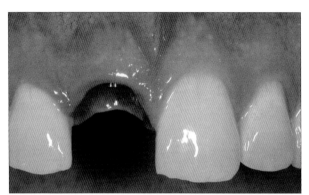

Fig 25b   Upon removal of the provisional and abutment, the peri-implant tissues were irrigated with air and water.

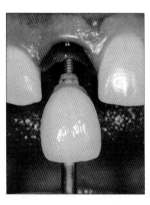

Fig 26a   Frontal view showing the seating of the crown onto the implant.

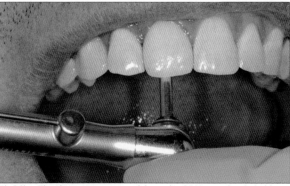

Fig 26b   The abutment screw was tightened to 35 Ncm and sealed with cotton and composite.

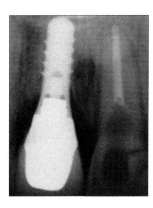

Fig 27   Periapical radiograph taken after insertion of the crown.

A periapical radiograph was taken and the patient was scheduled for a follow-up visit after three weeks (Fig 27).

At the three-week follow-up, the peri-implant tissue was examined and the occlusion checked (Fig 28).

Oral hygiene and home-care procedures were reviewed with the patient. The patient was scheduled for maintenance visits every six months.

Acknowledgments

Surgical Procedures

Dr. James Ruskin – Professor, University of Florida, USA, Center for Implant Dentistry

Laboratory Procedures

Mitchell Jim – M & M Dental Laboratory, Gainesville, Florida, USA

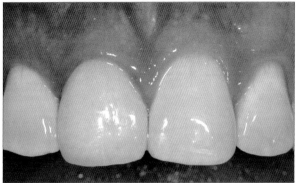

Fig 28   The three-week follow-up showed good tissue contours and excellent facial and interproximal tissue support.

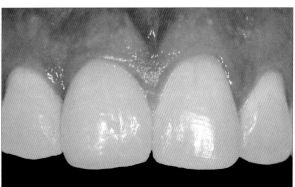

Fig 29a   Frontal view six months after insertion.

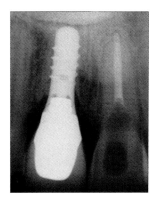

Fig 29b   Radiograph six months after insertion.

4.11 Replacement of an Upper Left Persisting Deciduous Canine with a Regular Neck Implant, Restored with a Ceramo-Metal Crown, Horizontally Screw-Retained

U. C. Belser

In October 1999, the 35-year-old female patient, a non-smoker, presented at our clinic with a persisting deciduous canine 63 that displayed all the clinical signs and symptoms of an ankylosed primary tooth, including inadequate crown volume, discoloration, locally perturbed occlusal plane, inharmonious course of the associated soft tissue, advanced root resorption, and increased mobility. The patient had a strong wish for a durable improvement of the situation with a clear emphasis on dental/gingival esthetics.

The patient was in good general health, and her medical history revealed no significant findings.

At full smile, the patient exhibited a high lip line, exposing all of the teeth and part of the gingiva (Fig 1).

The patient's gingival biotype was thin to medium thick and highly scalloped, presenting a broad band of keratinized mucosa (Fig 2).

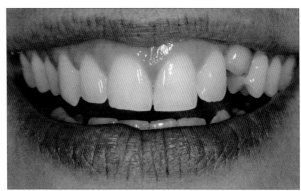

Fig 1   Full smile. High lip line revealing a significant portion of the gingiva. The persisting deciduous upper left canine was responsible for the severely disturbed symmetry of the anterior maxillary dentition, creating significant visual tension.

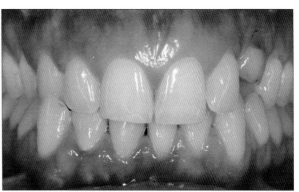

Fig 2   The thin to medium thick, highly scalloped gingival biotype increased the esthetic risk in this patient.

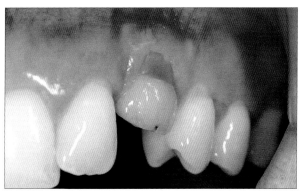

Fig 3   The band of keratinized mucosa associated with tooth 63 was narrow, and the free gingiva was located apically of that of the neighboring teeth.

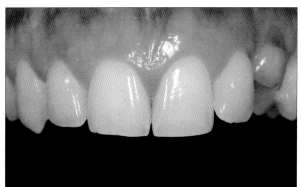

Fig 4   Disharmony in the tooth alignment caused by tooth 63.

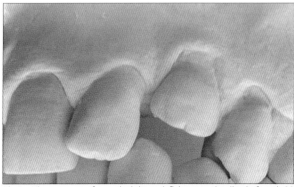

Fig 5   The presence of a vertical tissue deficiency to the distal of tooth 22 increased the esthetic risk.

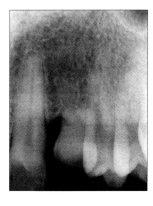

Fig 6   Pre-treatment periapical radiograph showing the extent of root resorption of tooth 63, vertical bone loss on the distal aspect of tooth 22, and the vertical bone volume available at the prospective implant site.

However, the keratinized gingiva was narrow at site 63 (Fig 3).

The harmony of the gingival margin line was disrupted by the persisting ankylosed deciduous canine, which also caused a marked disharmony in the alignment of anterior teeth (Fig 4).

The patient's clinical crowns tended towards a triangular shape, indicating an increased esthetic risk.

Except for tooth 63, the incisal edges of the maxillary incisors did not substantially differ in height compared to the respective contralateral teeth.

Clinical examination and periodontal probing revealed that vertical tissue deficiencies were present at sites 22 – 24, particularly to the distal of tooth 22, where the cemento-enamel junction (CEJ) was completely exposed (Fig 5).

The distance between the CEJ and the alveolar bone crest exceeded 3 mm. This recession further increased the esthetic risk, since more bone and, subsequently, soft tissue would be lost after the extraction of tooth 63 and flap elevation at the time of implant placement.

The periapical radiograph confirmed significant vertical tissue loss (bone and related soft tissue) distal of tooth 22, which would negatively affect the final esthetic treatment outcome. Beyond these findings, the clinical and radiographic examination did not reveal any signs of pathologic processes (Fig 6).

If the preoperative clinical and radiographic examination indicates that an implant-based solution cannot provide a "perfect illusion" from an esthetic point of view, the decision-making process should be extended to include a thorough analysis of available conventional prosthodontic alternatives. In this case, possible conventional prosthodontic alternatives to replace the missing tooth 23 included a three-unit resin-bonded ("Maryland") or ceramo-metal FPD, or eventually a "cantilever" FPD using teeth 24 and 25 as abutments. Since the lateral incisor cannot serve as an optimal bridge abutment either mechanically or esthetically and teeth 24 and 25 were virgin teeth, these options were rejected. The fact that both neighboring teeth were intact further supported the decision to insert a dental implant (Belser and coworkers, 2003; Belser and coworkers, 2004; Buser and coworkers, 2004; Higginbottom and coworkers, 2004).

The above findings led to the following esthetic risk profile (Table 1):

Table 1 The patient's individual esthetic risk profile

Esthetic Risk Factors	Low	Medium	High
Medical status	Healthy and cooperative patient, intact immune system		Reduced immune system
Smoking habit	Non-smoker	Light smoker (< 10 cig/d)	Heavy smoker (> 10 cig/d)
Patient's esthetic expectations	Low	Medium	High
Lip line	Low	Medium	High
Gingival biotype	Low scalloped, thick	Medium scalloped, medium thick	High scalloped, thin
Shape of tooth crowns	Rectangular		Triangular
Infection at implant site	None	Chronic	Acute
Bone level at adjacent teeth	≤ 5 mm to contact point	5.5 to 6.5 mm to contact point	≥ 7 mm to contact point
Restorative status of neighboring teeth	Virgin		Restored
Width of edentulous span	1 tooth (≥ 7 mm)	1 tooth (< 7 mm)	2 teeth or more
Soft-tissue anatomy	Intact soft tissue		Soft-tissue defects
Bone anatomy of alveolar crest	Alveolar crest without bone deficiency	Horizontal bone deficiency	Vertical bone deficiency

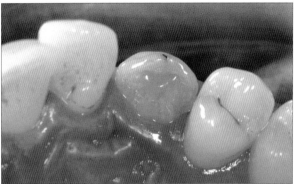

Fig 7 Adequate shade selection is an integral part of any routine prosthodontic procedure, including provisionals, which should match as closely as possible the shade of the neighboring natural dentition.

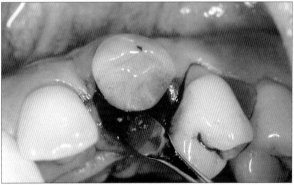

Fig 8 Situation before extraction, palatal view.

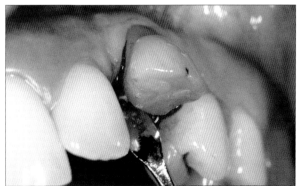

Fig 9 The deciduous tooth 63 could easily be mobilized with a small desmotome.

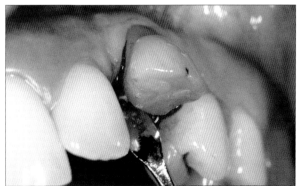

Fig 10 Care was taken to minimize trauma to the soft tissue.

This overall clinical situation can be classified as advanced to complex and is thus associated with a high esthetic risk.

Still at the first appointment, the shade for the removable provisional restoration was determined (Fig 7).

An intact reference tooth was defined for shade-taking. This is usually the contralateral tooth. Individual characteristics of the reference tooth, such as surface texture, should also be documented and communicated to the dental technician.

At the second appointment, the deciduous canine was carefully extracted (Figs 8 – 10).

Due to advanced root resorption, the deciduous tooth was easily removed by elevating it from the palatal aspect with a lancet-shaped desmotome, leaving the labial tissue basically untouched.

Also due to the root resorption, the alveolus was quite shallow (Fig 11).

This situation was considered advantageous for the establishment of primary stability in the apical region on implant placement.

The horizontal aspect of the bony arch was harmoniously contoured and did not have any major horizontal deficiencies. From a vertical viewpoint, however, the labial tissue deficiency was clearly visible (Fig 12).

No further "ridge preservation" procedures were performed at the time of extraction.

Immediately after the extraction, a provisional removable partial denture was inserted to maintain the patient's basic esthetic and phonetic functions (Fig 13).

At this stage, it was important to ensure that no significant tissue compression would occur. "Fit Checker" was used to identify pressure spots, which were subsequently removed. To align the provisional with the line of the neighboring natural teeth and the mucosa line, its pink base was also modified at insertion (Fig 14).

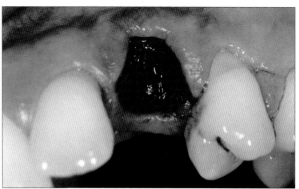

Fig 11   As anticipated from the radiograph and the clinical examination, the resulting extraction socket was shallow.

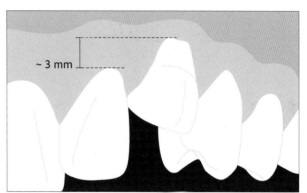

Fig 12   Soft-tissue conditions with a soft-tissue deficiency around tooth 63, creating an esthetic risk.

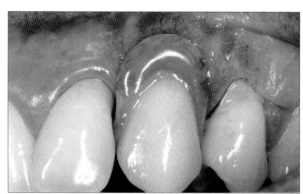

Fig 13   The transient removable partial denture helped maintain esthetics and phonetics.

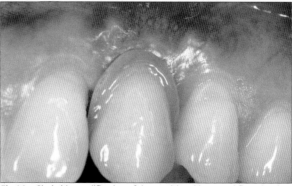

Fig 14   Chairside modification of the provisional improved fit and esthetics.

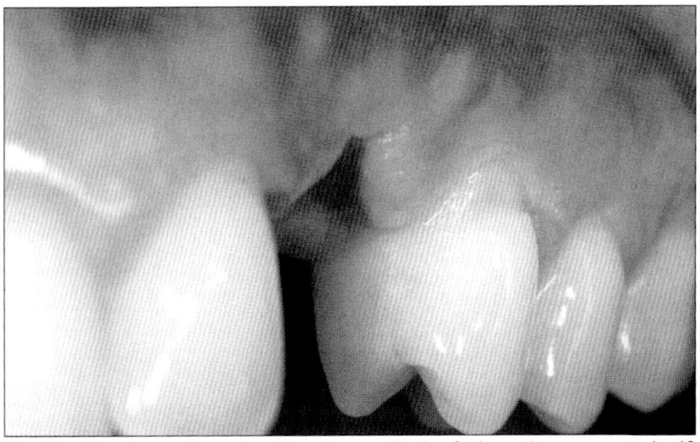

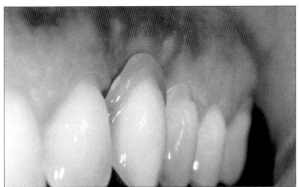

Fig 15   Ten days after extraction, the vertical soft-tissue loss was not significant.

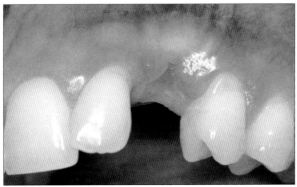

Fig 16   Moderate horizontal tissue loss had occurred since the extraction.

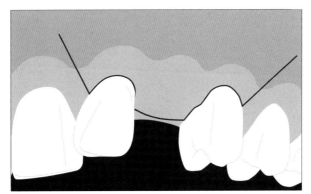

Fig 17   Status before implant placement.

Fig 18   The crestal incision was placed slightly palatally.

Ten days after extraction, the first phase of uneventful soft-tissue healing was completed. No significant vertical soft-tissue loss had taken place (Fig 15).

A more frontal view of the extraction site with the partial denture in place demonstrated moderate horizontal tissue loss (Fig 16)

Eight weeks after the extraction, soft-tissue healing was completed, and the patient was scheduled for the placement of a Standard implant (Fig 17).

A full-thickness flap was elevated in local anesthesia, including mesial and distal relieving incisions and a crestal incision located approximately 2 – 3 mm palatally (Fig 18).

The flap was extended through the sulcus of the adjacent teeth, ascending to the facial aspect of the alveolar crest with divergent distal line angle relieving incisions.

The mucoperiosteal flap was carefully raised, exposing the underlying alveolar bone (Fig 19).

After implant-bed preparation, which included minimal bone scalloping, a Standard Implant was placed (Fig 20).

The implant shoulder was located significantly more apically, approximately 2 mm apically of the CEJ of the neighboring teeth (Fig 21). This was necessary due to a significantly more apical location of the marginal bone in relation to the CEJ of the natural teeth. The full extent of the bone loss at tooth 22 was clearly visible.

In order to improve the thickness and contour of the labial bone plate, which should be at least 2 mm thick, the labial aspect of the implant site was augmented with a low-substitution bone substitute (Fig 21).

This augmentation procedure served to enhance long-term soft-tissue esthetics.

The implant was covered with a small closure screw (Fig 21). A free connective-tissue graft was harvested from the palatal premolar region at the time of implant placement. The connective-tissue graft was placed over the augmented implant site in a coronal position. It covered the coronal portion of the implant (Fig 22), improving the volume and position of the marginal tissue.

To avoid displacement of the graft and to ensure optimal vascularization, it was carefully sutured to the periosteum of the full-thickness flap.

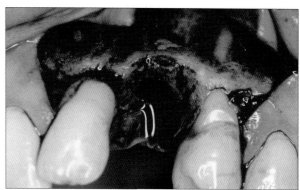

Fig 19 The bone allowed for secure primary stability.

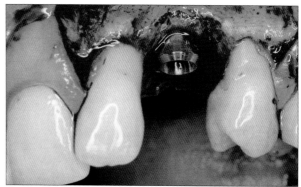

Fig 20 Slightly apical implant shoulder position due to the bony defect around tooth 12.

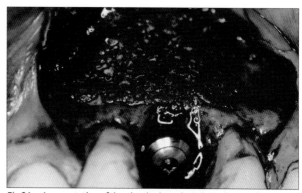

Fig 21 Augmentation of the alveolar bone in order to improve its contour – a prerequisite for optimal esthetics.

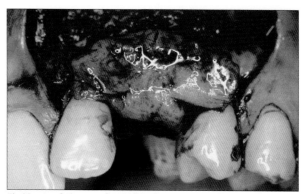

Fig 22 A soft-tissue graft was placed to compensate for the soft-tissue deficiency at site 23.

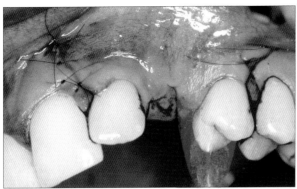

Fig 23   Tension-free wound closure facilitating uneventful soft-tissue healing.

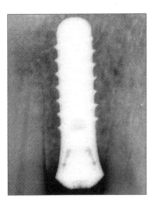

Fig 24   Periapical radiograph illustrating the slight apical position of the implant shoulder.

Following the incision of the periosteum, the flap was carefully mobilized coronally, precisely repositioned, and sutured free of tension with 6.0 non-resorbable suture material (Fig 23).

After implantation and soft-tissue grafting, a periapical radiograph was taken (Fig 24).

Seven days after implant placement, the site was inconspicuous (Fig 25), documenting successful soft tissue graft integration. The sutures could be removed.

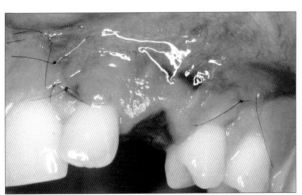

Fig 25   One week after implant placement.

After another six weeks, the site was re-entered to gain access to the coronal implant portion. The small closure screw was removed and replaced by a longer healing cap (Fig 26). This served to establish a soft-tissue "tunnel" from the implant to the oral cavity and initiated the soft-tissue conditioning phase.

To preserve precious keratinized mucosa, the tissue was opened with a scalpel instead of a tissue punch. A significant volume of keratinized soft tissue was moved to the mesial aspect of the implant site (Fig 26).

The tissue blanching caused by the pressure of the healing cap on the soft tissue indicated the start of the mucosa-conditioning process.

The restorative phase was initiated two weeks after the installation of the healing cap (Fig 27).

Seen from labially, the height of the soft-tissue margin at the implant site was now located more coronally than at the time of extraction of the deciduous canine (Figs 28, 29).

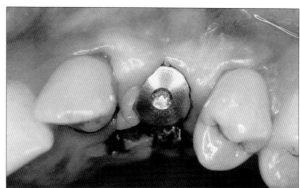

Fig 26 A healing cap was attached to establish and maintain a soft tissue "tunnel" which would provide easy access to the implant shoulder for the prosthetic procedures.

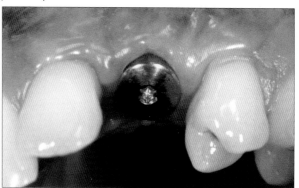

Fig 27 Uneventful healing of the soft tissues after installation of the healing cap.

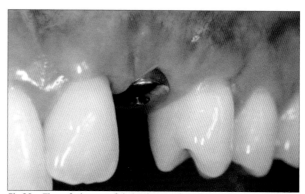

Fig 28 The soft-tissue graft helped move the soft-tissue margin at the implant site more incisally.

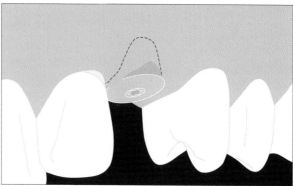

Fig 29 Soft-tissue margin before (red) and after (blue) the grafting procedure.

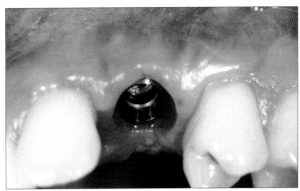

Fig 30   A stable epithelium.

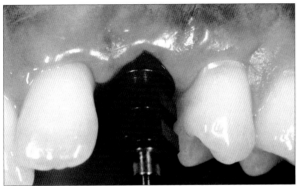

Fig 31   Connecting the impression cap. The soft tissue must not be damaged.

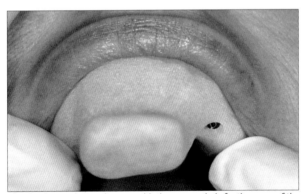

Fig 32   Custom impression tray with the passage hole for the screw of the impression cap.

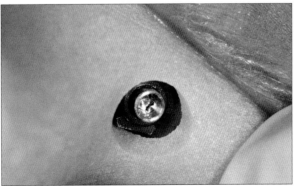

Fig 33   Easy access to the screw of the impression cap.

Once the healing cap was removed for impression taking, the first phase of the process leading to the establishment of a scalloped soft-tissue line was completed (Fig 30).

A screw-retained synOcta impression cap was connected to the implant shoulder and tightened with the integral guide screw (Fig 31). The custom impression tray was tried in to ensure a precise fit and easy access to the screw (Figs 32, 33).

The screw access hole of the impression cap was covered with wax to prevent it from being blocked by impression material and to ensure easy access (Fig 34).

A polyether impression was taken (Fig 35) and an implant analog fixed on the impression cap (Fig 36).

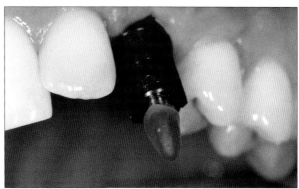

Fig 34   A wax cover for the screw facilitated easy loosening of the impression cap after the impression was taken.

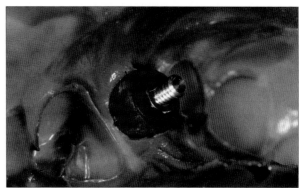

Fig 35   Apical view of the impression cap, ready for connection of the implant analog.

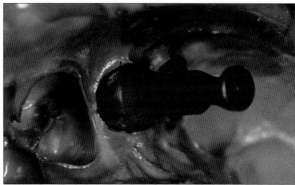

Fig 36   The implant analog was attached to the impression cap and secured with the respective screw before the master cast was made.

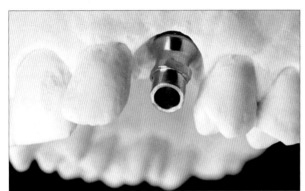

Fig 37   The post for the temporary crown needed to be shortened.

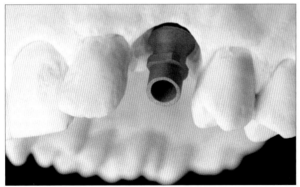

Fig 38   The post was shortened to the desired occlusal height.

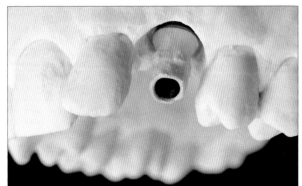

Fig 39   Sandblasting facilitated adhesion of the opaque.

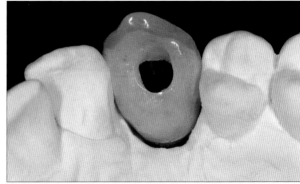

Fig 40   Applying the opaque.

Fig 41   The screw channel must not interfere with the occlusion.

A stone cast was produced for the fabrication of a transocclusally screw-retained provisional composite crown. The crown was fabricated on the basis of a titanium synOcta post for temporary restorations (Fig 37).

The post was shortened to the desired length (Fig 38), sandblasted (Fig 39), and coated with opaque (Fig 40).

The temporary implant-supported restoration was completed using a traditional composite-layering technique (dentine and enamel, using composite of different shades and levels of opacity), based on a previously generated waxup and a derived silicone guide. The implant axis was ideal, so the screw access opening was located at the palatal aspect of the crown, which in this manner could be screw-retained transocclusally (Fig 41).

A long interproximal contact line was established to compensate for the vertical soft-tissue deficiency distal of tooth 22 to reduce the size of the interproximal black triangles (Figs 42, 43).

Looking from the incisal aspect, the design of these "wings" becomes more apparent (Fig 44).

At the time of the integration of the provisional crown, the soft-tissue blanching occurring at insertion (Fig 45) indicated that volume had been added at the cervical portion of the restoration. This additional volume was necessary to achieve harmony with the emergence profiles of the natural adjacent teeth.

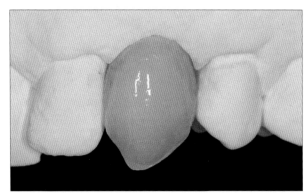

Fig 42   Provisional crown, labial view.

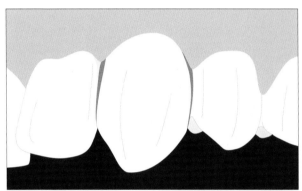

Fig 43   Long interproximal contacts compensated for interproximal soft-tissue deficiencies.

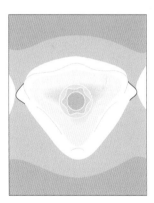

Fig 44   The long interproximal contacts were located slightly more palatally.

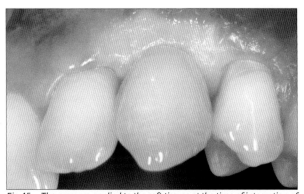

Fig 45   The pressure applied to the soft tissues at the time of integration of the provisional crown initiated the soft-tissue conditioning phase.

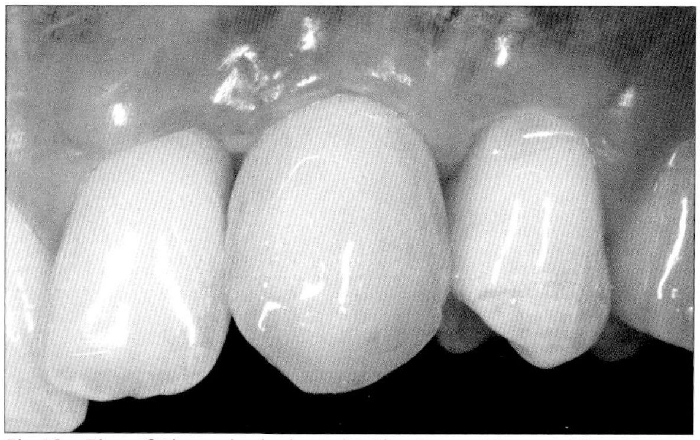

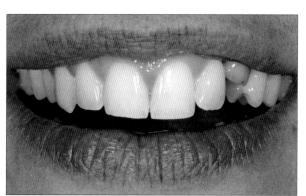

Fig 46   The soft tissues had adapted to the shape of the provisional crown.

One week after insertion of the provisional crown, the mucosa had adapted to the shape of the provisional (Fig 46). The incisal portion had been slightly modified to comply with the patient's esthetic expectations.

In the region of the mesial papilla, the dehiscence at the distal aspect of tooth 22 was clearly visible, as expected, leading to a slight disharmony in the marginal mucosa line.

Compared to the initial situation in October of 1999 (Fig 47a), esthetics had been significantly improved (Fig 47b).

Before the insertion of the final implant-supported superstructure, the peri-implant soft tissue had to present optimal three-dimensional contours. The soft-tissue conditioning process usually takes three to six months.

The provisional crown remained in situ for three months to create optimal contours. At that point, the decision was made to proceed with the final restoration.

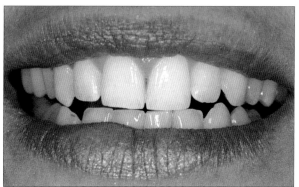

Fig 47a   Before treatment.

Fig 47b   After insertion of the provisional crown.

In the dental laboratory, a synOcta transversal (TS) abutment for transversally screw-retained crowns was selected and placed on the implant analog (Fig 48).

This approach provided more room in the incisal third of the restoration. This made it possible to avoid impairment of the optical properties of the more incisal regions of the final crown, such as translucency of the screw-access channel. Furthermore, the screw-access channel did not interfere with dynamic occlusion.

In order to permit perfect positioning of the respective metal component, the peri-implant soft tissue had to be modified at its palatal aspect: The model was relieved to generate space for positioning the cervical portion of the crown carrying the screw-retention part (Fig 49).

The ceramo-metal crown was fabricated according to a standard protocol: A metal framework based on a prefabricated cast-on component was created and veneered with compatible ceramics, applying a complex layering technique to achieve the required optical properties (Figs 50 – 52).

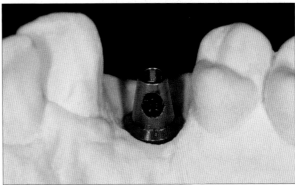

Fig 48   A TS abutment was attached to the implant analog.

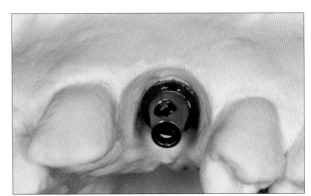

Fig 49   TS abutment on the analog, incisal view

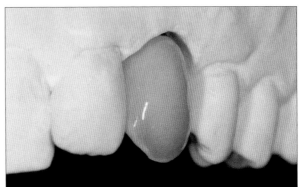

Fig 50   The final crown, labial view.

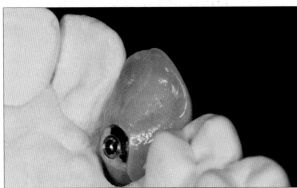

Fig 51   Transversal screw in the cervical portion of the crown, palatal view.

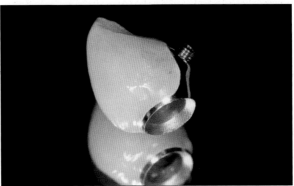

Fig 52   The crown and the small-sized transversal screw.

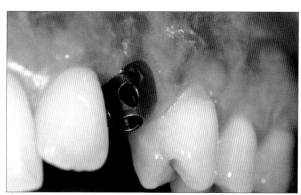

Fig 53   The abutment was inserted before the integration of the implant-supported transversally screw-retained crown.

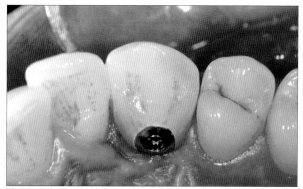

Fig 54   Palatal view of the final implant restoration showing easy access for manipulating the transversal screw. The screw-access channel was protected by a minimal perimeter of metal.

Before the insertion of the final ceramo-metal crown, the abutment was tightened to 35 Ncm (Fig 53).

The crown was attached to the abutment and the transversal screw tightened to 15 Ncm (Fig 54).

The implant-supported crown blended in well with the natural dentition in an esthetically pleasing way, matching the natural teeth in shape, texture, and color. The course of the marginal gingiva and the lines of the incisal edges were harmonious and esthetically appealing (Figs 55 – 57).

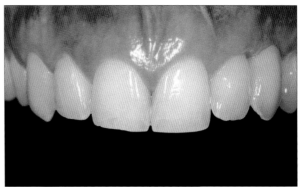

Fig 55   Clinical appearance immediately after installation of the final crown.

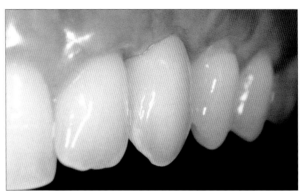

Fig 56   A more tangential view. Straight vestibular emergence profile of the implant-supported restoration, establishing harmony with the buccal contour of the adjacent natural dentition.

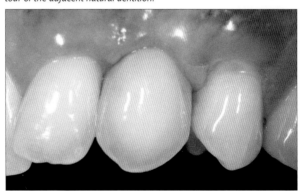

Fig 57   The implant-supported superstructure blended in nicely with the natural dentition.

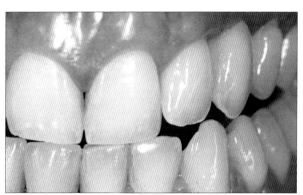

Fig 58   The occlusal guidance during lateral excursion of the mandible was meticulously checked, and any interference was carefully removed.

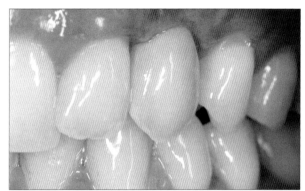

Fig 59   The cervical position of the screw access channel helped create a disturbance-free occlusion.

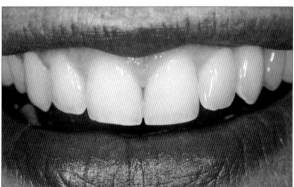

Fig 60   The patient was satisfied with the esthetic treatment outcome.

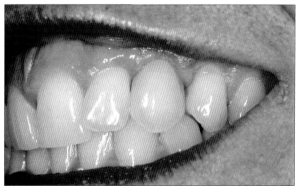

Fig 61   Stable soft tissue conditions twelve months after final crown installation.

The occlusion was carefully checked. Minor discrepancies were adjusted (Figs 58, 59).

The patient's smile after insertion of the final crown is seen in Figures 60 and 61. She was very pleased with the esthetic treatment outcome.

The situation twelve months after integration of the final restoration is seen in Figure 61.

The periapical radiograph twelve months after implant placement shows a stable bone level (Fig 62).

At the five-year clinical follow-up in March 2005, the soft-tissue contours as well as the bone contours were stable (Figs 63 – 65).

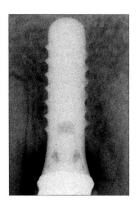

Fig 62 Stable bone contours twelve months after final crown installation.

Acknowledgments

Surgical Procedures
Dr. Daniel Buser – Professor, University of Bern, Switzerland, Department of Oral Surgery and Stomatology

Laboratory Procedures
Master Dental Technician Michel Magne – Oral Design Montreux, Switzerland

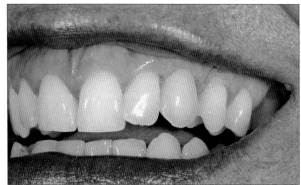

Fig 63 Five years after insertion of the crown, the peri-implant soft tissues continued to be stable.

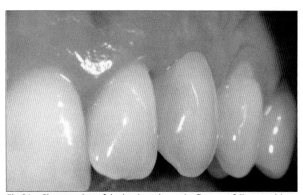

Fig 64 Close-up view of the implant site at the five-year follow-up visit.

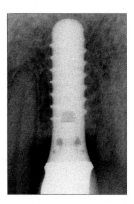

Fig 65 Five-year periapical radiograph showing a stable bone level around the dental implant.

4.12 Replacement of a Congenitally Missing Upper Left Lateral Incisor with a Narrow Neck Implant, Restored with a Ceramo-Metal Crown, Transocclusally Screw-Retained

B. Schmid

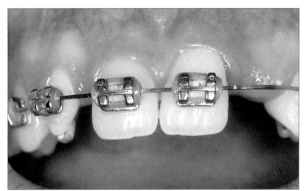

Fig 1   Clinical situation at baseline (1999), frontal view.

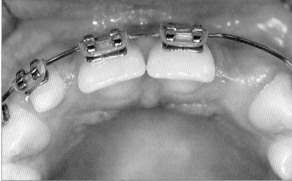

Fig 2   Clinical situation at baseline, incisal view.

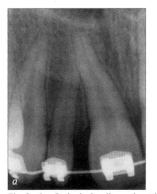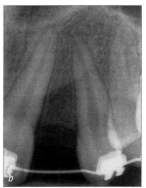

Figs 3a, b   Periapical radiographs at baseline. Widening of the gap in position 22 as well as root parallelization were necessary before implantation.

An 18 year-old female patient, a non-smoker, presented in 1999 during orthodontic treatment with a tooth gap in position 22 due to a congenitally missing permanent tooth 22 and a peg-shaped permanent tooth 12 (Figs 1–3).

Orthodontic treatment had started four years before, when the patient was 14 years old, to correct a complex situation by maxillary expansion in combination with a bracket treatment. The patient had been referred by the orthodontist for clarification of a possible implant therapy to define the ideal size of the tooth gap at site 22 as well as the necessary root parallelization for implant placement, i.e. final minor orthodontic corrections to create an ideal situation for implant placement.

During the remainder of the orthodontic treatment, tooth 12 was brought to a position that would allow for the placement of an esthetically pleasing laminate veneer, giving the tooth crown a shape that would blend in well with the line of natural teeth. The size of the gap at site 22 was adjusted to approximately 6 mm for the placement of a Narrow Neck (NN) implant (Figs 4, 5).

The patient wanted the gap at site 22 closed and the shape of tooth 12 improved. She had high esthetic expectations with regard to the treatment outcome.

Before implant placement, a ceramic laminate veneer was bonded to the peg-shaped tooth 12 (Figs 6, 7).

After the veneering procedure, the placement of a NN implant in site 12 was planned.

The periapical radiograph taken after orthodontic treatment demonstrated the straightened tooth axes of teeth 21 and 23 and the widened gap, which now had a mesiodistal width of approximately 6 mm (Fig 8).

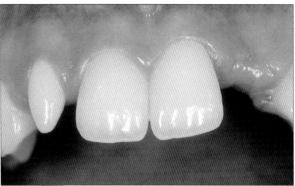

Fig 4   Clinical situation after orthodontic treatment, frontal view.

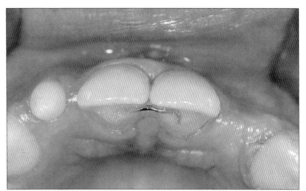

Fig 5   Clinical situation after orthodontic treatment, with retainers, incisal view.

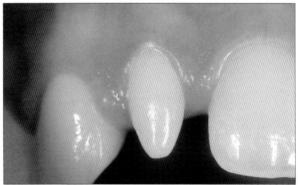

Fig 6   Ideal position of tooth 12 for the bonding of a ceramic laminate veneer, thanks to orthodontic alignment.

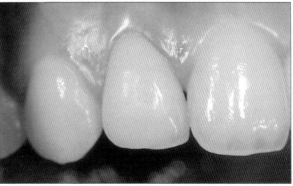

Fig 7   Tooth 12 two months after the bonding of the ceramic laminate veneer.

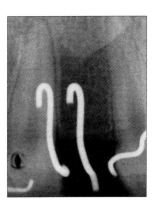

Fig 8   Periapical radiograph of the future implant site after orthodontic treatment. The wires of the retainers and the wires of the removable partial denture to close the gap at site 22 were visible.

Radiologically, the interproximal bone-crest levels at teeth 21 and 23 were well maintained, allowing for a distance of less than 5 mm between the contact points of the future crowns and the interproximal bone-crest (Tarnow and coworkers, 1992; Choquet and coworkers, 2001) (Fig 8). Periodontal probing confirmed this radiological finding and delivered probing depths of 2 mm around teeth 21 and 23.

The patient's smile line was medium high, displaying all of the tooth crowns and marginal soft tissue at full smile. The tissue biotype was thin and highly scalloped. The shape of the tooth crowns tended towards the triangular.

The clinical and radiological findings in combination with the patient's esthetic treatment expectations led to an esthetic risk profile summing up to a medium esthetic risk (Table 1).

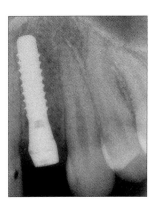

Fig 9   Situation after implant placement.

Based upon the above analysis, a treatment plan was drawn up, preparing for the placement of a Standard Plus implant with a NN prosthetic platform (Ø 3.5 mm) and a length of 12 mm length in semi-submerged healing mode. The implant axis was planned in a way that would allow for transocclusal screw retention of the future superstructure.

Due to an apical fenestration defect at the time of implant placement caused by the horizontal bone deficiency, a simultaneous augmentation procedure was performed. This also allowed for the optimization of the horizontal bone volume and contour. Good primary stability and an ideal three-dimensional implant position were achieved (Figs 9, 10).

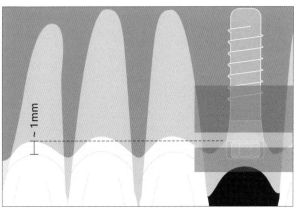

Fig 10   The implant shoulder was located in the apicocoronal comfort zone.

Table 1 The patient's individual esthetic risk profile.

Esthetic Risk Factors	Low	Medium	High
Medical status	Healthy and cooperative patient, intact immune system		Reduced immune system
Smoking habit	Non-smoker	Light smoker (< 10 cig/d)	Heavy smoker (> 10 cig/d)
Patient's esthetic expectations	Low	Medium	High
Lip line	Low	Medium	High
Gingival biotype	Low scalloped, thick	Medium scalloped, medium thick	High scalloped, thin
Shape of tooth crowns	Rectangular		Triangular
Infection at implant site	None	Chronic	Acute
Bone level at adjacent teeth	≤ 5 mm to contact point	5.5 to 6.5 mm to contact point	≥ 7 mm to contact point
Restorative status of neighboring teeth	Virgin		Restored
Width of edentulous span	1 tooth (≥ 5.5 mm)	1 tooth (< 5.5 mm)	2 teeth or more
Soft-tissue anatomy	Intact soft tissue		Soft-tissue defects
Bone anatomy of alveolar crest	Alveolar crest without bone deficiency	Horizontal bone deficiency	Vertical bone deficiency

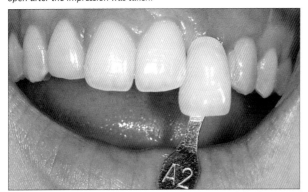

Fig 11   Clinical situation eight weeks after implant placement. A gingivectomy was performed and a longer healing cap was placed to keep the space open after the impression was taken.

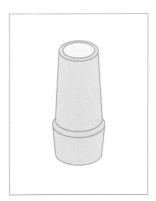

Fig 12   As in most young patients, A2 was the best match for the natural tooth color.

Fig 13   NN titanium coping.

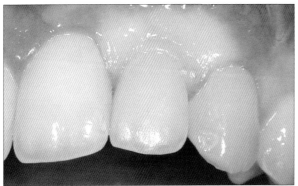

Fig 14   Pressure needs to be applied to the peri-implant mucosa to start the soft-tissue conditioning process.

Eight weeks after implant placement, the soft tissues were healthy and had healed well (Fig 11). It was therefore decided to take an impression to enable fabrication of a provisional restoration.

Before taking the impression, the appropriate tooth shade was determined (Fig 12).

A NN coping, titanium, was used for the fabrication of a provisional cement-retained crown (Fig 13).

At the time of delivery of the provisional crown, a distinct blanching of the mucosa was visible due to the pressure applied by the provisional (Fig 14).

The provisional was given its ideal shape at the time of integration, and adaptations of the provisional crown during the course of the mucosa-conditioning process were set aside. This explains the extent of blanching. Due to this initial compression of the soft tissue, some patients request an anesthesia for this step of the treatment. The blanching of the mucosa should disappear within 10 to 15 minutes.

Because of the patient's young age, the provisional crown could have been left in situ for a time (one year or more) to avoid discrepancies in incisal-edge positions. Continued skeletal growth might then lead to a change in the positions of the natural teeth, whereas the implant position would remain stable. This might lead to discrepancies in the vertical position of the incisal edges (Bernard and coworkers, 2004).

Nine months after loading with the provisional crown, the desired emergence profile was well developed (Fig 15) so that it was decided to take the impression for the final crown (Fig 16).

In the dental laboratory, a master cast was poured for the fabrication of the final ceramo-metal crown, with the emergence profile precisely matching the anatomy of the conditioned mucosa.

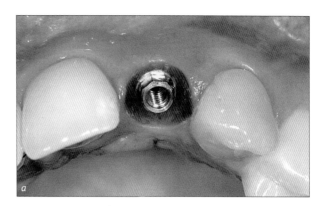

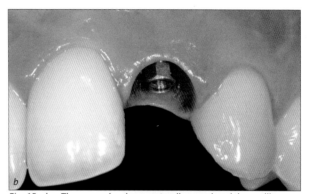

Figs 15a, b   The mucosal arch was naturally curved, and the papillae were well shaped.

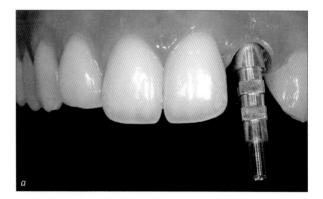

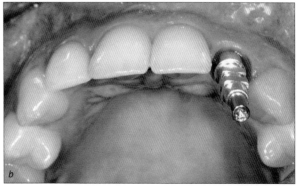

Figs 16a, b   A NN impression cap was screw-tightened on the implant shoulder.

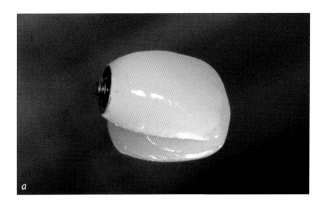

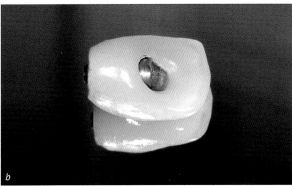

Figs 17a, b   *The final transocclusally screw-retained ceramo-metal crown ready for insertion.*

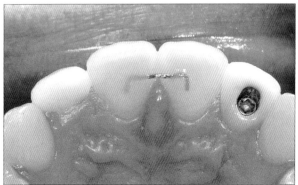

Fig 18   *Situation after tightening of the occlusal screw at 35 Ncm, ready for sealing the screw access hole.*

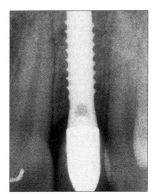

Fig 19   *The crown was precisely seated on the implant shoulder.*

The implant axis had been planned to "exit" through the dental cingulum of the planned restoration, which made transocclusally screw-retained attachment mode possible (Fig 17a). The crown was fabricated using an NN framework blank made from an oxidizable alloy not suitable for casting-to, which was directly veneered with veneering ceramics (Fig 17b).

After integration of the final crown, the occlusion was checked to detect and remove possible disturbances. The crown was cleaned and the screw-access channel sealed with composite material (Fig 18).

The periapical radiograph taken after loading with the final crown confirmed the exact fit of the crown on the implant shoulder (Fig 19).

B. Schmid

In 2004, two years after crown insertion, the follow-up periapical radiograph confirmed stable peri-implant bone-crest levels (Fig 20).

At the same visit, the peri-implant tissues were inspected. Facial and interproximal tissue support was ideal, with excellent soft-tissue stabilization (Fig 21).

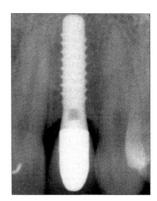

Fig 20 Two-year follow-up radiograph.

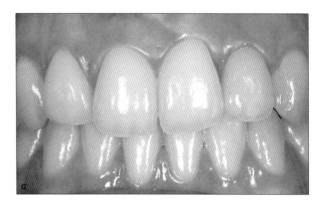

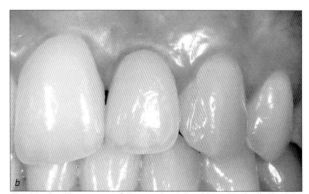

Figs 21a, b The two year follow-up showed stable and esthetically pleasing soft-tissue contours.

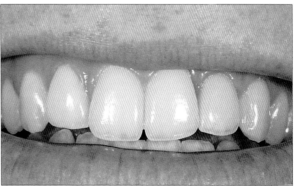

Fig 22 The dental esthetics at full smile were excellent.

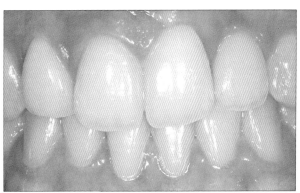

Fig 23   Frontal view 3½ years after prosthetic rehabilitation.

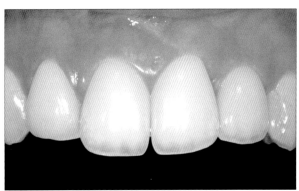

Fig 24   Close-up at 3½ years.

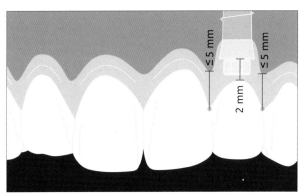

Fig 25   Due to the ideal relations of implant shoulder, bone crest, and contact points, the soft tissue was stable.

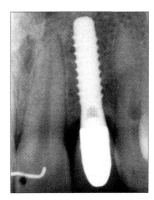

Fig 26   3½-year follow-up radiograph.

The smile-line photograph documented the pleasing and stable esthetic treatment outcome (Fig 23).

At the beginning of 2006, 3½ years after crown insertion, the peri-implant soft tissue continued to be stable (Fig 23).

The close-up photograph 3½ years after loading with the final crown confirmed the pleasing and stable esthetic treatment outcome (Figs 24, 25).

The 3½-year periapical radiograph confirmed stable bone crest levels (Fig 26).

Acknowledgments

Orthodontic pre-treatment
Dr. Philipp Schnyder – Bern, Switzerland

Surgical Procedures
Dr. Daniel Buser, Professor, University of Bern, Switzerland, Department of Oral Surgery and Stomatology

Laboratory Procedures
Master Dental Technician Beat Heckendorn – Bern, Switzerland

4.13 Replacement of Congenitally Missing Upper Lateral Incisors with Narrow Neck Implants, Restored with Ceramo-Metal Crowns, Cemented

W. C. Martin

A healthy 19-year-old male patient presented at our clinic for a consultation on treatment options to replace the congenitally missing teeth at sites 12 and 22 (Fig 1). He expected the treatment to be performed within one year, as he was planning to move away from the area.

After a consultation on treatment options, the patient requested an implant-retained fixed restorative solution. A detailed examination of the teeth and periodontium adjacent to the edentulous spaces was performed to assess the potential for an esthetic result (Figs 2a-d).

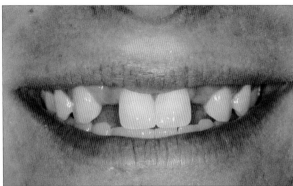

Fig 1   At full smile, the patient presented with a medium lip line, displaying the incisal and middle thirds of the clinical crowns and the tips of the papillae

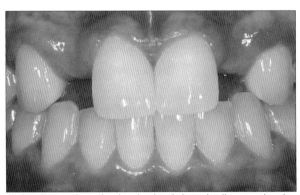

Fig 2a   Retracted anterior view showing virgin teeth adjacent to the edentulous spaces and a medium gingival biotype with moderate scalloped papillae and medium-thick tissue. A thin band of keratinized tissue spanned the area from canine to canine.

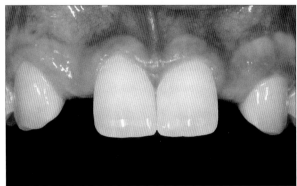

Fig 2b   Open-retracted view showing square-shaped teeth and irregular gingival margins between the canines and central incisors. Inadequate clinical crown exposure on tooth 23. The excess tissue height was favorable, as it allowed for modifications during the surgical procedures.

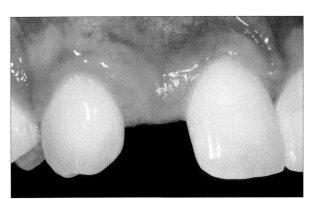

Fig 2c   Open-lateral of teeth 13 and 11. Excess tissue height in the edentulous space, indicating a potential need for hard-tissue scalloping during implant placement to allow for proper vertical positioning of the implant shoulder. Probing depths were 2 mm around teeth 13 and 11.

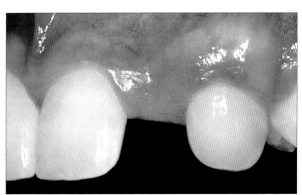

Fig 2d   Open-lateral view of teeth 21 and 23. Excess tissue height in the edentulous space as well as on the facial side of tooth 23. The surgical procedures planned would address excess tissue problem. Probing depths were 2 mm around teeth 21 and 23.

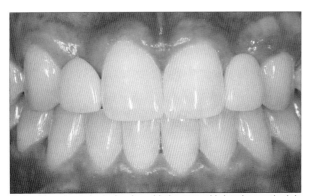

Fig 3   The retracted anterior view with the removable interim prosthesis in place. Confirmation of the edentulous span (7 mm) was possible as the denture teeth were acceptable in size and shape.

The patient reported that orthodontic therapy had recently been completed and that the edentulous spaces were maintained with an interim removable prosthesis (Fig 3).

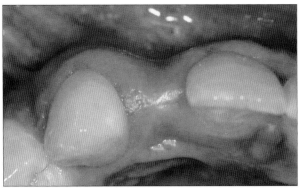

Fig 4a   Occlusal view of the edentulous space at site 12, revealing a horizontal hard-tissue deficiency.

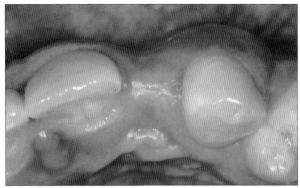

Fig 4b   Occlusal view of the edentulous space at site 22, revealing a horizontal hard-tissue deficiency.

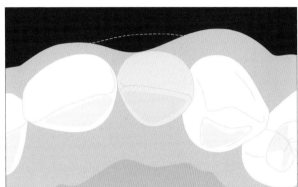

Fig 4c   Horizontal deficiency at site 22 with the proposed restoration place.

Close inspection of the denture teeth on the interim restoration indicated that adequate facial and interproximal tissue height existed to allow for tooth replacement with soft-tissue margins symmetrical to those of adjacent teeth. It was also apparent that the horizontal tissue thickness was inadequate to allow for a pleasant-looking "root-form" emergence of the definitive restorations. The occlusal view without the prosthesis in place confirmed these horizontal deficiencies (Figs 4a-c).

Figure 4c with the proposed future restoration in place explains the need for a bone-augmentation procedure to address the horizontal bone deficiencies.

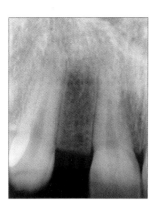

Fig 5a   Periapical radiograph of site 12. Interproximal root space less than 7 mm, alveolar crest less than 5 mm from the desired contact point.

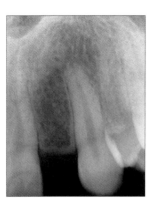

Fig 5b   Periapical radiograph of site 22. Interproximal root space less than 7 mm, alveolar crest height less than 5 mm from desired contact point.

Examination of the periapical radiographs revealed ideal space between the roots of the adjacent teeth as well as an ideal height of the interproximal crests for papilla support (Figs 5a-b).

An examination of the panoramic radiograph revealed several potential donor sites for hard tissue, if any was needed for grafting procedures (Fig 6).

Consideration was given to the patient's age and predicted completion of growth. Unable to obtain serial lateral cephalographs, the best determinant of growth completion, a hand-wrist film was used to examine the fusion of the epiphysis and diaphysis of the middle phalanx and the degree of calcification of the ulnar sesamoid bone (Proffit and coworkers, 1992) (Fig 7). In general, male patients above the age of 19 are good candidates for implant therapy. Risks associated with premature implant placement include delayed passive eruption of the anterior dentoalveolar segments and orthodontic relapse of the adjacent teeth with subsequent "intrusion" of the implant restorations. A correction will most often require replacement of the restoration or orthodontic retreatment.

After the consultation, the data obtained were compiled for the esthetic risk-assessment table (Table 1):

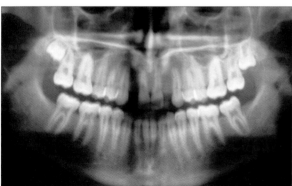

Fig 6   The panoramic radiograph revealed potential donor sites in the ramus and chin areas.

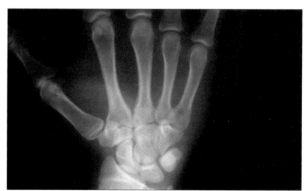

Fig 7   A view of the hand-wrist film depicting fusion of the epiphysis and diaphysis of the middle phalanx and the degree of calcification of the ulnar sesamoid bone.

Table 1 The patient's individual esthetic risk profile.

Esthetic Risk Factors	Low	Medium	High
Medical status	Healthy and cooperative patient, intact immune system		Reduced immune system
Smoking habit	Non-smoker	Light smoker (< 10 cig/d)	Heavy smoker (> 10 cig/d)
Patient's esthetic expectations	Low	Medium	High
Lip line	Low	Medium	High
Gingival biotype	Low scalloped, thick	Medium scalloped, medium thick	High scalloped, thin
Shape of tooth crowns	Rectangular		Triangular
Infection at implant site	None	Chronic	Acute
Bone level at adjacent teeth	≤ 5 mm to contact point	5.5 to 6.5 mm to contact point	≥ 7 mm to contact point
Restorative status of neighboring teeth	Virgin		Restored
Width of edentulous span	1 tooth (≥ 5.5 mm)	1 tooth (< 5.5 mm)	2 teeth or more
Soft-tissue anatomy	Intact soft tissue		Soft-tissue defects
Bone anatomy of alveolar crest	Alveolar crest without bone deficiency	Horizontal bone deficiency	Vertical bone deficiency

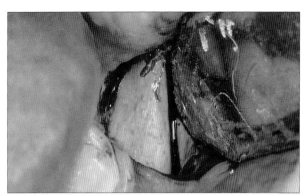

Fig 8a   A vertical releasing incision to expose the lateral border of the ramus.

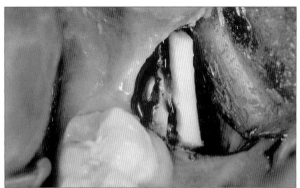

Fig 8b   A straight fissure carbide bur was used to create a vertical section in the lateral portion of the ascending ramus.

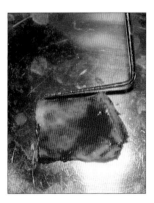

Fig 8c   A 1.5 × 1.5 cm harvested donor block.

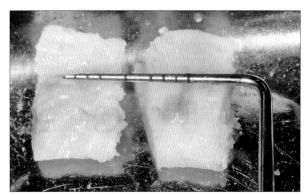

Fig 8d   Two 7 × 7 mm blocks created from the donor block to be used for onlay grafting at sites 12 and 22.

Taking into consideration the patient's age, virgin adjacent teeth, and desire for long-term function, dental implants and restorations were chosen. The overall esthetic risk for this treatment was low. This low esthetic risk indicated that the potential for an esthetic result based upon the ITI Consensus Statements (Belser and coworkers, 2004) for an implant restoration was high. With this favorable diagnosis, a comprehensive treatment plan was drawn up to treat these edentulous sites with an expedited approach. Three phases of treatment were planned:

1. Augmentation – Bilateral autogenous hard tissue grafts were to be placed to enhance width.
2. Surgery – In a restoration-driven approach, two Narrow Neck (NN) Implants were to be placed.
3. Restorative – Provisional and final restorations were to be fabricated to enhance form, function, and esthetics.

Autographs and allographs were considered. Due to the patient's limited available treatment time, bilateral autogenous ramus graphs were indicated. A 1.5 × 1.5 cm donor block graft was harvested from the left ramus and sectioned into two 7 × 7 mm blocks (Figs 8a-d).

A mid-crestal and a distal vertical releasing incision were executed, followed by a periosteal releasing incision. The periosteal releasing incision allowed for placement of the donor block and membrane, followed by tension-free closure (Figs 9a-p).

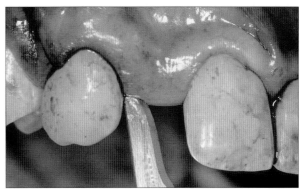

Fig 9a   A mid-crestal incision at site 12 performed with a straight #12 blade.

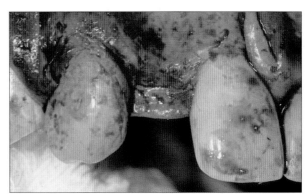

Fig 9b   Elevation of the tissue and removal of any soft-tissue residue on the surface of the bone.

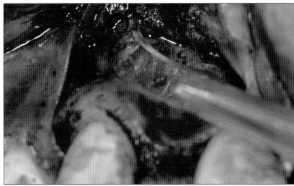

Fig 9c   Periosteal releasing incision performed with a curved #15c blade.

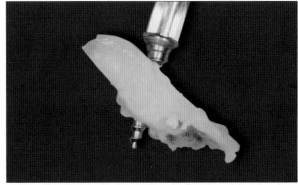

Fig 9d   After the donor block was adjusted to fit to the recipient site, a bone screw was placed in it to simplify intraoral placement.

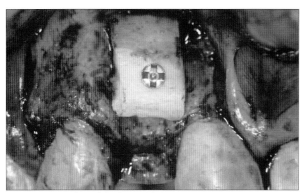

Fig 9e   Frontal view of the fixated block.

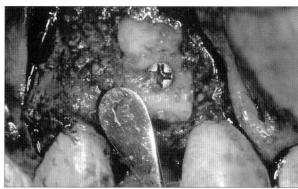

Fig 9f   Cancellous bone collected during the preparation procedures was packed around the block before covering it with the membrane.

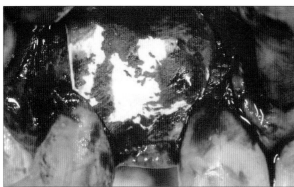

Fig 9g   Placement of a resorbable membrane.

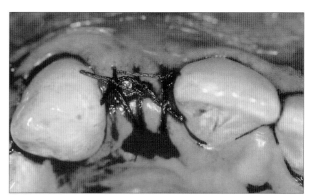

Fig 9h   Occlusal view after suturing.

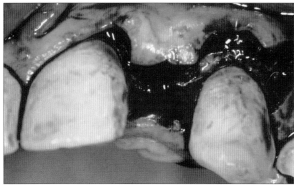

Fig 9i   A mid-crestal incision at site 22 performed with a straight #12 blade.

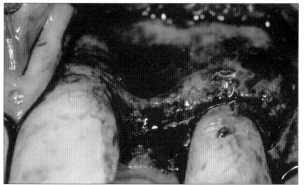

Fig 9j   Elevation of the tissue and removal of any soft-tissue residue on the surface of the bone.

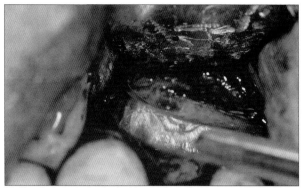

Fig 9k   Periosteal releasing incision performed with a curved #15c blade.

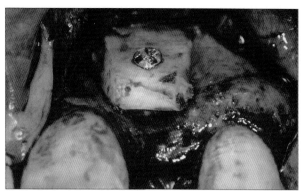

Fig 9l   Occlusal view of the fixated block.

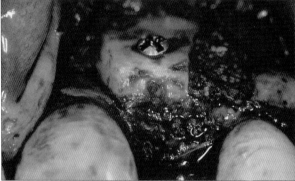

Fig 9m   Cancellous bone collected during the preparation procedures was packed around the block before covering it with the membrane.

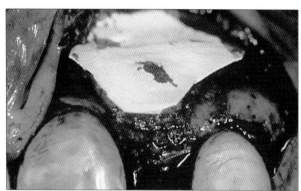

Fig 9n   Placement of a resorbable membrane.

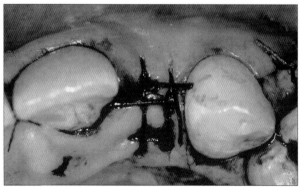

Fig 9o   Occlusal view after suturing.

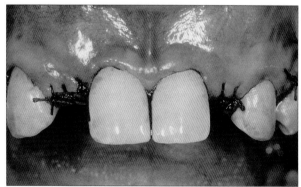

Fig 9p   Frontal postoperative view.

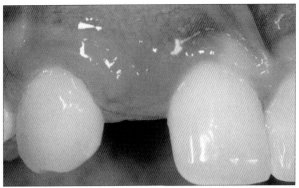

Fig 10a Lateral view of edentulous site 12, three months after grafting.

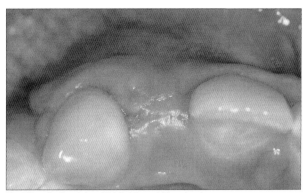

Fig 10b Occlusal view highlighting width gained.

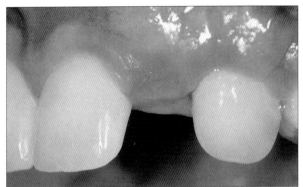

Fig 10c Lateral view of edentulous site 22, three months after grafting.

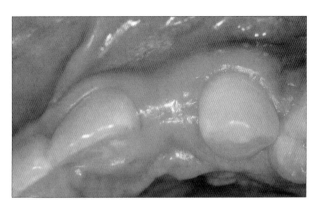

Fig 10d Occlusal view highlighting width gained.

At the completion of surgery, the removable interim partial denture was adjusted to create space between the denture teeth and the incision lines. The patient was placed on antibiotics (amoxicillin 500 mg three times a day for seven days) and a mouth-rinse (chlorhexidine). He was also instructed to eat a soft diet and to avoid situations that would create pressure on the graft sites. The sutures were removed at the follow-up visit one week later.

After three months of healing, the patient returned for a presurgical workup. Diagnostic casts were poured to perform a waxup and to fabricate surgical templates (Figs 10a-d). In the laboratory, the diagnostic waxup was performed highlighting the proposed soft-tissue margin position of the implant restorations was utilized to assist in planning the ideal implant position (Figs 11a-f).

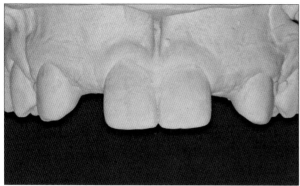

Fig 11a   Frontal view of the diagnostic cast.

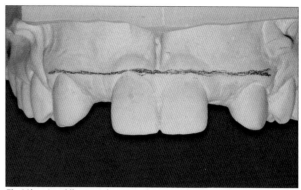

Fig 11b   A red line was drawn on the cast to indicate a harmonious gingival margin spanning from tooth 13 to tooth 23.

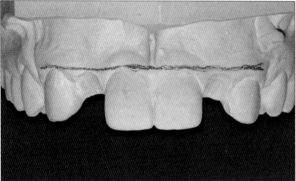

Fig 11c   Excess soft/hard tissue height ne-cessitated a scalloping procedure on the cast to al-low proper placement of the soft-tissue margin of the proposed implant restoration.

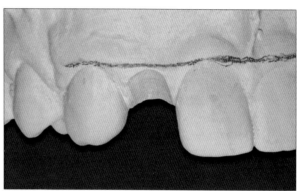

Fig 11d   Lateral view of site 12 highlighting the scalloping performed to place the soft-tissue margin slightly superior to the red line connecting the gingival margins of teeth 13 and 11.

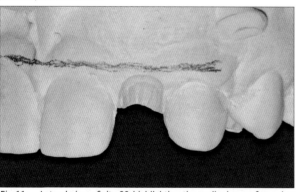

Fig 11e   Lateral view of site 22 highlighting the scalloping performed to place the soft-tissue margin slightly superior to the red line connecting the gingival margins of teeth 21 and 23.

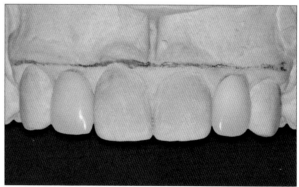

Fig 11f   Frontal view of the diagnostic waxup.

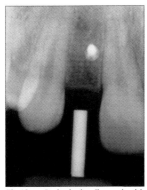

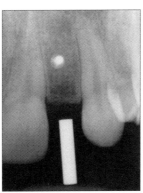

Fig 12a   Periapical radiograph with the radiographic template in place.

Fig 12b   Periapical radiograph with the radiographic template in place.

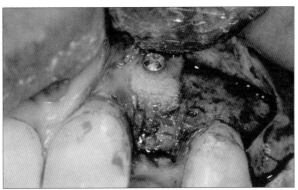

Fig 13   Minimal tissue reflection allowing access to the titanium retaining screw at site 22.

Once the planned restorations were determined, a radiographic template was fabricated for surveying before the fabrication of the surgical template (Figs 12a, b). The template utilized a rod 10 mm in length and 2.2 mm in diameter and indicated the proposed implant position. Coronal tissue thickness and radiographic distortion could be accounted for based on the known dimensions of the rod. This assisted the surgeon in selecting the ideal implant length for the site.

Upon confirmation of the radiographic survey, the surgical template was fabricated. At the time of surgery, a minimal tissue reflection was performed to obtain access to the retaining screw (Fig 13). A 0.5 mm template (vertical template) highlighting the proposed mucosal margin of the implant restoration was placed. Scalloping of the osseous crest was performed to allow for the placement of the implant shoulder approximately 2 mm apical of the zenith of the vertical template (Figs 14a, b).

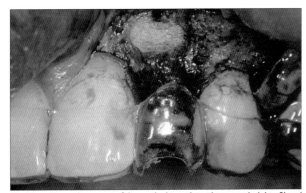

Fig 14a   Upon placement of the vertical template, the excess height of hard tissue can be appreciated.

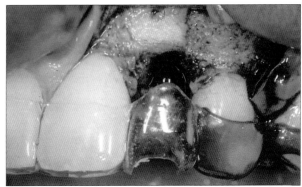

Fig 14b   After scalloping. Osseous crest located at a position that allows for the vertical placement of the dental implant shoulder, 2 mm apically of the proposed mucosal restorative margin.

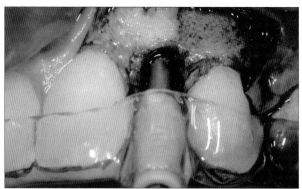

Fig 15a   Initial preparation through the drill sleeve with a small round bur.

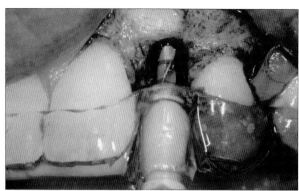

Fig 15b   Preparation through the drill sleeve with a 2.2-mm twist drill to a depth of 12 mm.

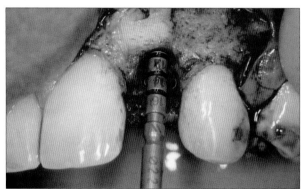

Fig 15c   Confirmation of the initial depth of the osteotomy with the 2.2-mm alignment pin.

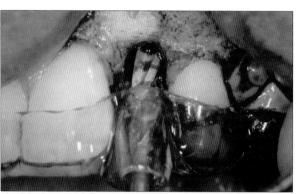

Fig 15d   Removed drill sleeve. Preparation with the 2.8-mm twist drill to a depth of 12 mm.

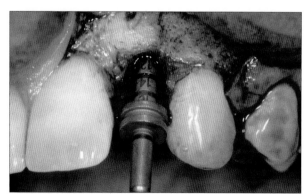

Fig 15e   Confirmation of osteotomy depth and angulations with the 2.8-mm depth gauge.

Once the hard tissue scalloping was completed, a 1.0 mm template with drill sleeve was placed that allowed for the preparation of the osteotomy site while directing orofacial and mesiodistal angulations (Figs 15a-e). The site was prepared for a Narrow Neck implant 12 mm in length. Upon completion of the osteotomy, the implant was placed with close regard to the vertical position of the shoulder.

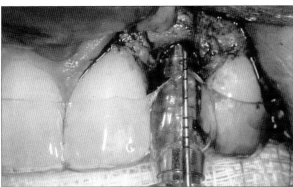

Fig 16a   Before the removal of the transfer post, the vertical depth of the implant was confirmed using the vertical template.

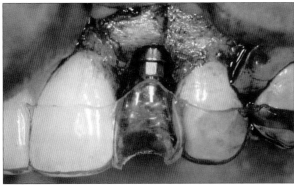

Fig 16b   After the removal of the transfer post, the implant shoulder was clearly visible up to the zenith of the template.

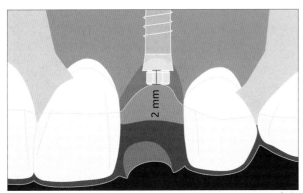

Fig 16c   Final distance from the implant shoulder to the planned soft-tissue margin of the restoration (2 mm).

Before the removal of the transfer post, the vertical template was used to help confirm the proper implant depth (Figs 16a-c).

After removal of the transfer post, the healing cap was placed and the tissue closed with a 4-0 vicryl suture (Figs 17a, b). The patient was sent for a postoperative radiograph while the interim restoration was adjusted to prevent contact with the healing cap under function (Fig 18). The patient was scheduled for a follow-up appointment after one week.

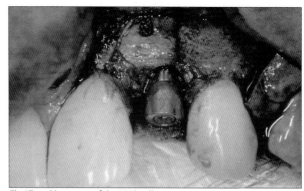

Fig 17a   Placement of the NN healing cap.

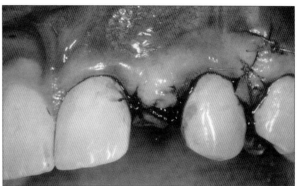

Fig 17b   After surgical suturing.

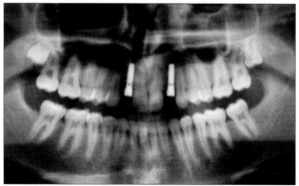

Fig 18   Postoperative panoramic radiograph confirming final implant angulations.

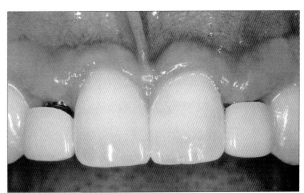

Fig 19a   Six weeks after implant placement.

Six weeks after implant placement, the patient was scheduled for a loading visit (Figs 19a-e). At that appointment, provisional restorations were fabricated that would initiate maturation of the transition zone. As mentioned in Chapter 1.2, the transition zone is the emergence created from the shoulder of the implant to the soft-tissue margin.

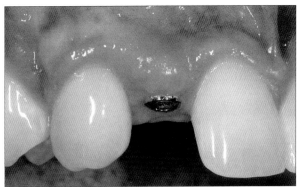

Fig 19b   Lateral view of implant 12 implant six weeks after implant placement.

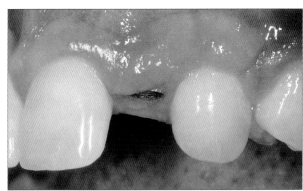

Fig 19d   Lateral view of implant 22 six weeks after implant placement.

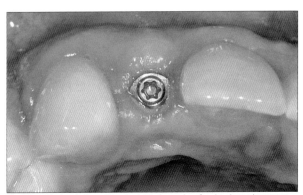

Fig 19c   Occlusal view of implant 12 six weeks after implant placement.

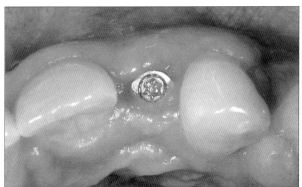

Fig 19e   Occlusal view of implant 22 six weeks after implant placement.

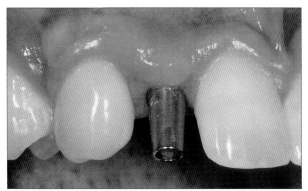

Fig 20a   NN titanium coping in place on implant 12. A high-speed carbide bur was used to mark indicator grooves (mid-facial, interproximal, palatal, and gingival) to assist with extraoral preparation.

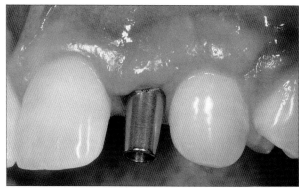

Fig 20b   NN titanium coping in place on implant 22. A high-speed carbide bur was used to mark indicating grooves (mid-facial, interproximal, palatal, and gingival) to assist with extraoral preparation.

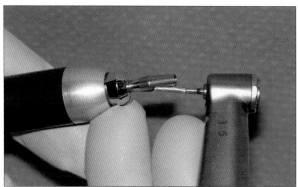

Fig 20c   Extraoral preparation of the titanium coping using the analog holder.

After placement of the NN titanium copings on the implants and tightening to 15 Ncm, indicator grooves were prepared on the surface with a high-speed carbide bur to help obtain the correct reduction and angulations while the definitive finishing was performed extraorally (Figs 20a-d). In general, titanium should not be prepared intraorally in order to avoid impregnating the tissue with titanium particles.

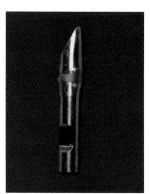

Fig 20d   Final preparation design of the titanium coping.

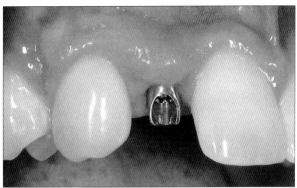

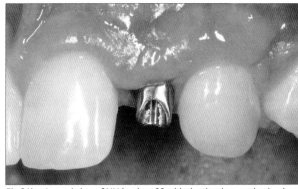

Fig 21a   Lateral view of the NN implant 12 with the titanium coping in place. The access hole was covered with cotton, and a polycarbonate crown was relined over it.

Fig 21b   Lateral view of NN implant 22 with the titanium coping in place. The access hole is covered with cotton, and a polycarbonate crown was relined over it.

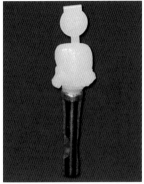

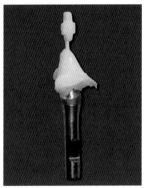

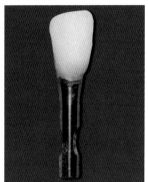

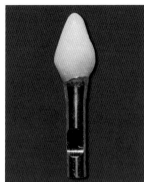

Fig 22a   Facial view of provisional crown 12 on the titanium coping and laboratory analog after the relining procedure.

Fig 22b   Lateral view of provisional crown 12 on the titanium coping and laboratory analog after the relining procedure.

Fig 23   Composite resin was added to the interproximal surfaces to create support for the peri-implant tissue, supporting the papillae.

Fig 24   Composite resin was added facially and palatally to create ideal emergence of the provisional restoration. Facially, the point at which the emergence becomes convex establishes the mucosal margin.

Once the custom preparation was complete, the copings were placed on the implants and the access holes blocked with cotton before the prefabricated polycarbonate crowns were relined (Figs 21a, b).

Once the provisionals had set intraorally, they were removed along with the copings and placed onto laboratory analogs (Figs 22a, b). Composite resin was added to create an emergence profile from the coping margin to the contact point, establishing the transition zone. Creating interproximal emergence requires straight or slightly convex support from the coping margin through the tissue to the contact point (Fig 23). The facial emergence contour was straight or concave from the coping margin to the proposed position of the mucosal margin, at which point it becomes convex (Fig 24). This convexity will help establish the final position of the mucosal margin of the implant restoration.

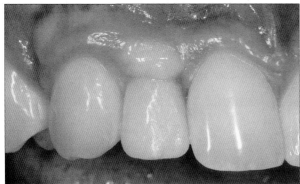

Fig 25a   Tissue blanching immediately after the placement of the provisional on implant 12.

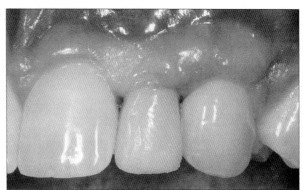

Fig 25b   Tissue blanching immediately after the placement of the provisional on implant 22.

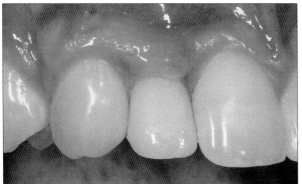

Fig 26a   Reduction in blanching noticed after 10 minutes.

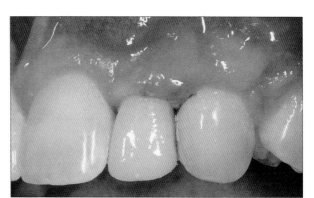

Fig 26b   Reduction in blanching noticed after 10 minutes.

Once the emergence modifications of the provisionals were completed, the copings were placed back on the implants, tightened to 15 Ncm, covered with cotton, and the provisionals were seated. Blanching of the tissue is often evident (Figs 25a, b). In general, if the blanching subsides within 10 minutes, no reduction in the emergence profile or removal of tissue is necessary (Figs 26a, b).

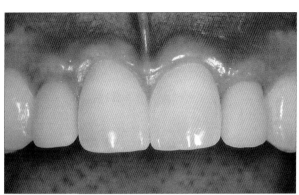

Fig 27a   Open-anterior view of the provisional restorations for teeth 12 and 22, four weeks after loading.

A return visit was scheduled for four weeks later, when a final impression was to be taken and the correct shade selected (Figs 27a-c).

In general, if dental bleaching is planned, it is performed during the 4-week tissue-maturation phase. After removal of the provisionals and copings, the tissue maturation in the transition zone can be appreciated (Fig 28).

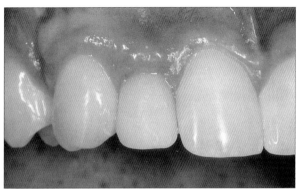

Fig 27b   Lateral view of the provisional restoration for tooth 12, four weeks after loading.

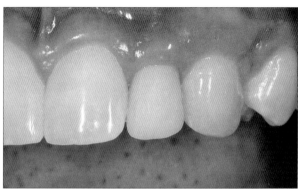

Fig 27c   Lateral view of the provisional restoration for tooth 22, four weeks after loading.

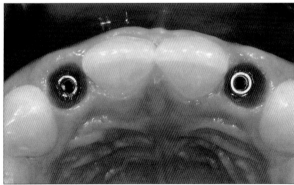

Fig 28   Occlusal view of implants highlighting the transition zone created by the provisionals.

Before the final impression, the shade was taken using photographs and communicated to the laboratory. NN snap-on impression caps were placed on the implants and a polyvinyl siloxane impression was made (Fig 29).

In the laboratory, NN laboratory analogs were inserted into the final impression, into which a low-expansion die stone was then poured (Figs 30a, b).

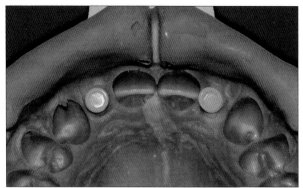

Fig 29 The polyvinyl siloxane impression with NN snap-on impression caps.

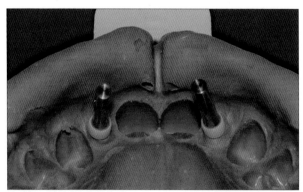

Fig 30a NN laboratory analogs were snapped into the impression caps.

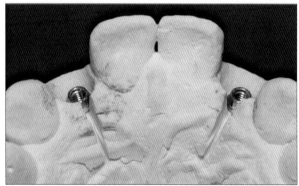

Fig 30b Master cast for fabrication of final copings and restorations.

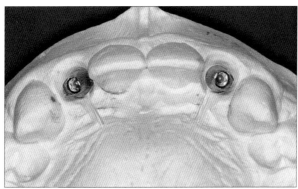

Fig 31a   Occlusal view of the titanium copings after preparation.

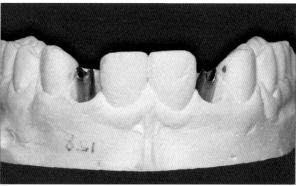

Fig 31b   Facial view of the titanium copings after preparation.

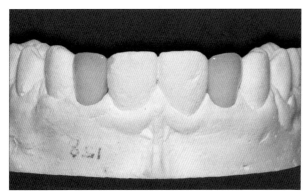

Fig 31c   Facial view of the ceramo-metal restorations on the titanium copings.

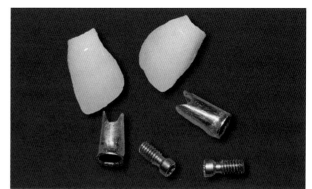

Fig 31d   Final restorations and customized copings as returned from the laboratory.

Two new NN titanium copings were used to fabricate the final custom copings and ceramo-metal restorations (Figs 31a-d).

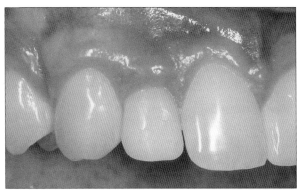

Fig 32a Lateral view of the provisional restoration for tooth 12 six weeks after loading.

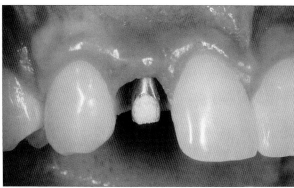

Fig 32b Lateral view of the coping and tissue support after removal of the provisional restoration for tooth 12.

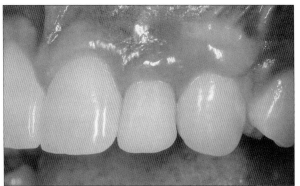

Fig 32c Lateral view of the provisional restoration for tooth 22 six weeks after loading.

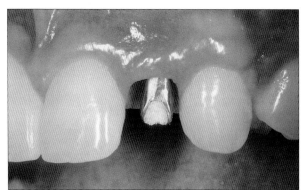

Fig 32d Lateral view of the coping and tissue support after removal of the provisional restoration for tooth 22.

At the delivery visit two weeks after the final impression had been taken, the provisional restorations and copings were removed (Figs 32a-d).

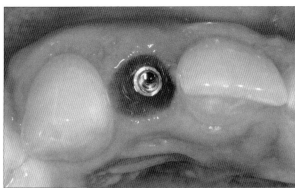

Fig 33a   Occlusal view of implant 12 after irrigation and before the insertion of the definitive coping. The transition zone was mature.

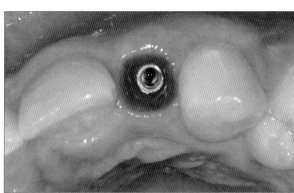

Fig 33b   Occlusal view of implant 22 after irrigation and before the insertion of the definitive coping. The transition zone was mature.

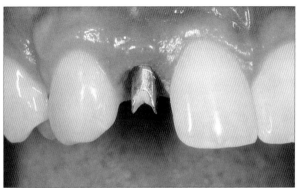

Fig 34a   After insertion of the definitive customized titanium coping for tooth 12, torqued to 35 Ncm, and sealed with cotton and Cavit.

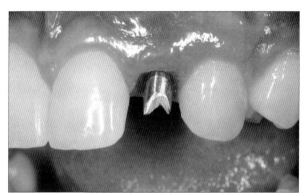

Fig 34b   After insertion of the definitive customized titanium coping for tooth 22, torqued to 35 Ncm, and sealed with cotton and Cavit.

The implants were irrigated with an air-water syringe before inserting the definitive copings (Figs 33a, b).

Once the fit and shade of the final restorations were confirmed, the coping screws were tightened to 35 Ncm. The screw access hole was covered with a cotton pellet and sealed with Cavit (3M Espe) (Figs 34a, b).

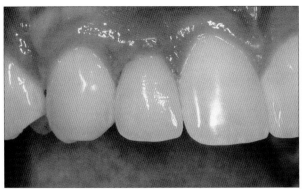

Fig 35a   Final restoration after delivery.

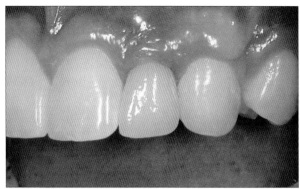

Fig 35b   Final restoration after delivery.

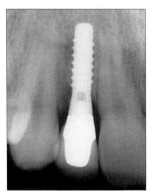

Fig 36a   Periapical radiograph of implant 21 after insertion of the final restoration.

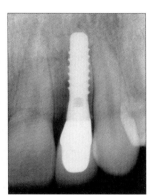

Fig 36b   Periapical radiograph of implant 22 after insertion of the final restoration.

The final restorations were cemented with a permanent cement and the occlusion was adjusted to a light shim-stock pull (Figs 35a, b). Adjustments to the ceramic surface were followed by a polishing procedure with diamond-impregnated discs that help to create a glaze-like surface on the ceramic.

Periapical radiographs were taken and the patient was scheduled for a three-week follow-up (Figs 36a, b).

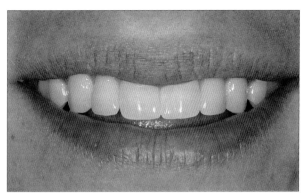

Fig 37a   Full smile, one year after insertion.

At the three-week visit, the peri-implant tissues were examined for cement residue, and the occlusion was checked. Oral hygiene and home-care procedures were reviewed with the patient. At the end of the visit, the patient was scheduled for yearly maintenance procedures. The patient was seen at the follow-ups at one year and two years (Figs 37a-n).

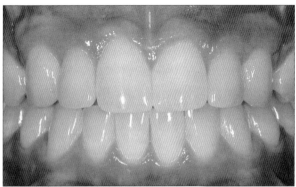

Fig 37b   Retracted view, one year after insertion.

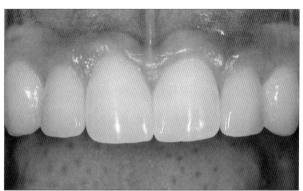

Fig 37c   Open-anterior view of teeth 12 and 22, one year after insertion.

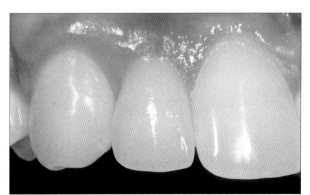

Fig 37d   Lateral view of tooth 12, one year after insertion.

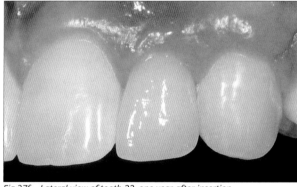

Fig 37f   Lateral view of tooth 22, one year after insertion.

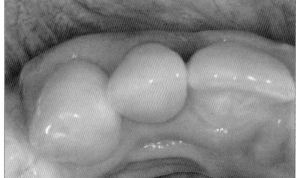

Fig 37e   Occlusal view of tooth 12, one year after insertion.

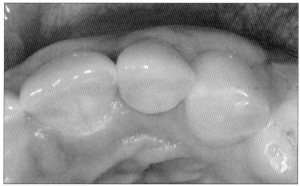

Fig 37g   Occlusal view of tooth 22, one year after insertion.

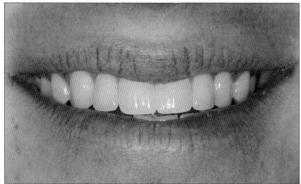

Fig 37h   Full smile, two years after insertion.

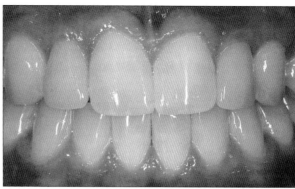

Fig 37i   Retracted view, two years after insertion.

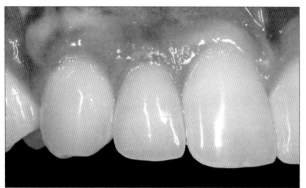

Fig 37j   Lateral view of tooth 12, two years after insertion.

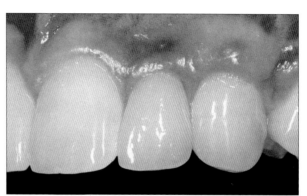

Fig 37k   Lateral view of tooth 22, two years after insertion.

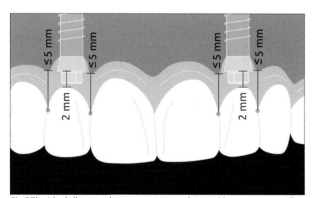

Fig 37l   Ideal distances between contact points and bone crest as well as between implant shoulders and soft-tissue margins. These help to ensure long-term stable esthetic treatment results.

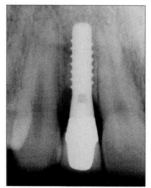

Fig 37m   Periapical radiograph of implant 12, two years after insertion.

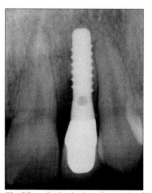

Fig 37n   Periapical radiograph of implant 22, two years after insertion.

Acknowledgments

Surgical Procedures
Dr. James Ruskin – Professor, University of Florida, USA, Center for Implant Dentistry

Laboratory Procedures
Mitchell Jim – M & M Dental Laboratory, Gainesville, Florida, USA

4.14 Replacement of an Upper Right Lateral Incisor with a Narrow Neck Implant, Restored with a Ceramo-Metal Crown, Cemented

W. C. Martin

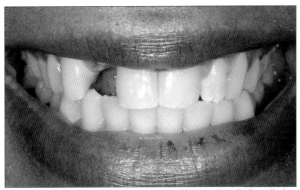

Fig 1   At full smile, the patient presented with a medium lip line, displaying the incisal and middle thirds of the clinical crowns and the tips of the papillae.

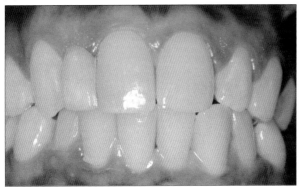

Fig 2   Retracted anterior view showing discolored teeth adjacent to the edentulous space, a medium gingival biotype with moderately scalloped papillae and medium-thick tissue. A moderate band of keratinized tissue spanned from canine to canine.

A healthy 32-year-old female patient presented at the clinic for recementation of a resin-retained fixed partial denture (RRFPD) and for a consultation on treatment options to replace the congenitally missing tooth 12 (Fig 1). She desired a more esthetic and functional treatment option than her current one.

A detailed examination of the teeth and periodontium adjacent to the edentulous space was performed to assess the esthetic risk for implant therapy. The intraoral exam revealed a pre-existing metal-reinforced RRFPD replacing tooth 12. Discoloration of teeth 13 and 11 due to the large metal retainers on the prosthesis was evident. The patient reported several occasions on which the prosthesis had debonded and had to be reinserted. It had become a nuisance for her, and she wanted a more permanent solution. Upon comparison of the adjacent lateral incisors, the mesiodistal width of 12 was slightly smaller and 22 was slightly undercontoured in its incisal embrasure (Fig 2).

Pontic 12 was a ridge-lap design masking the excessive tissue height in the edentulous space, indicating a sufficient amount of tissue for facial and interproximal support. It also indicated a potential need for hard-tissue scalloping during implant placement to allow for proper vertical positioning of the implant shoulder (Fig 3).

Adequate horizontal tissue thickness existed to allow for good "root-form" emergence of the proposed implant restoration (Fig 4). Probing depths were 2 mm circumferentially around teeth 13 and 11.

Examination of the periapical radiograph revealed limited space between the roots of the adjacent teeth as well as adequate height of the interproximal crests for papilla support (Fig 5).

After the consultation, the data obtained were compiled for the esthetic risk-assessment table (Table 1).

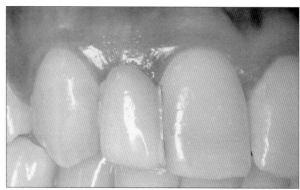

Fig 3 Lateral view revealing square-shaped teeth and harmonious gingival margins between the canine and central incisor. Broad contact points were evident at the retainers for tooth 12, which explained the esthetic problem.

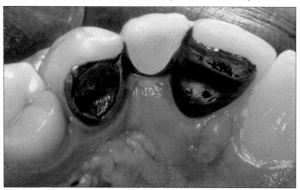

Fig 4 An occlusal view from tooth 13 to tooth 11 showing the large metal retainers used in the resin-retained restoration.

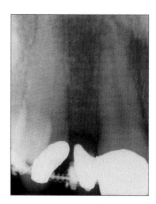

Fig 5 Periapical radiograph of site 12. Interproximal root space less than 7 mm, alveolar crest height less than 5 mm from the desired contact point.

Table 1   The patient's individual risk profile.

Esthetic Risk Factors	Low	Medium	High
Medical status	Healthy and cooperative patient, intact immune system		Reduced immune system
Smoking habit	Non-smoker	Light smoker (< 10 cig/d)	Heavy smoker (> 10 cig/d)
Patient's esthetic expectations	Low	Medium	High
Lip line	Low	Medium	High
Gingival biotype	Low scalloped, thick	Medium scalloped, medium thick	High scalloped, thin
Shape of tooth crowns	Rectangular		Triangular
Infection at implant site	None	Chronic	Acute
Bone level at adjacent teeth	≤ 5 mm to contact point	5.5 to 6.5 mm to contact point	≥ 7 mm to contact point
Restorative status of neighboring teeth	Virgin		Restored
Width of edentulous span	1 tooth (≥ 5.5 mm)	1 tooth (< 5.5 mm)	2 teeth or more
Soft-tissue anatomy	Intact soft tissue		Soft-tissue defects
Bone anatomy of alveolar crest	Alveolar crest without bone deficiency	Horizontal bone deficiency	Vertical bone deficiency

Taking into consideration the patient's previous experience with the RRFPD, its unesthetic appearance, and expectations for long-term support and function, a dental implant and restoration was chosen. The overall esthetic risk for this treatment is low. This low esthetic risk indicates that the potential for an esthetic result for an implant restoration is high based upon the ITI Consensus Statements (Belser and coworkers, 2004). With this favorable diagnosis, a comprehensive treatment plan was generated to treat the edentulous site with a comprehensive team approach. Three phases of treatment were planned:

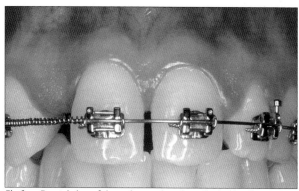

Fig 6a   Frontal view of the spring used on the orthodontic wire to create mesiodistal space.

1. Orthodontics—limited orthodontics would be done to create equal lateral spaces and to level out the incisal plane.
2. Surgery—utilizing a restoration-driven approach, a Narrow Neck (NN) implant would be placed.
3. Restorative—a provisional would be fabricated in addition to a final restoration focusing on form, function, and esthetics.

Orthodontics

The mesiodistal space at site 12 was enlarged orthodontically by approximately 1 mm (Figs 6a, b).

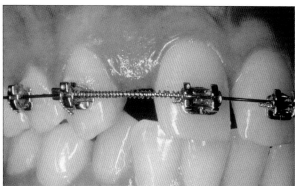

Fig 6b   Lateral view of site 12 during the orthodontic procedures.

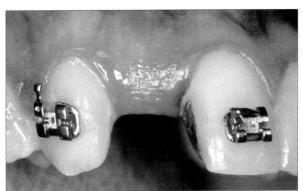

Fig 7a   Lateral view of site 12. 7 mm of mesiodistal space was created.

The pre-treatment dimension of site 12 was 6 mm, and of tooth 22, 7 mm. If desired, a denture tooth could be bonded to a bracket and incorporated into the orthodontic archwire, providing esthetics while tooth movement occurs. Upon completion of the orthodontic treatment, the patient was seen before the removal of the brackets to confirm that ideal restorative space was generated (Figs 7a-c).

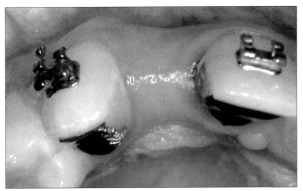

Fig 7b   Occlusal view of site 12 shows good width compared to the adjacent teeth.

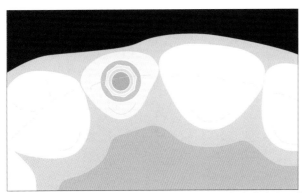

Fig 7c   Proposed axial implant position exiting through the incisal edge of the planned restoration.

Before the removal of the braces, the patient returned for a data-collection visit, during which diagnostic casts were fabricated. A diagnostic waxup was completed in the laboratory and a radiographic template fabricated (Figs 8a-d).

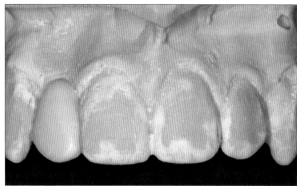

Fig 8a   Diagnostic waxup for a restoration-driven plan for implant placement.

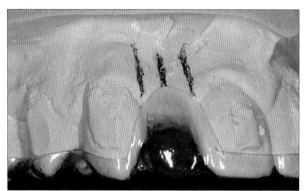

Fig 8b   A Vacuform template of the diagnostic waxup.

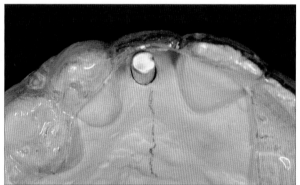

Fig 8c   Planning the implant position for a cement-retained restoration; the axis of implant placement exited through the incisal edge.

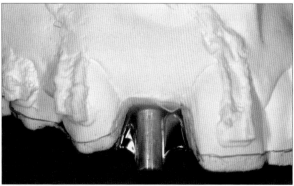

Fig 8d   Radiographic template on the duplicated diagnostic cast.

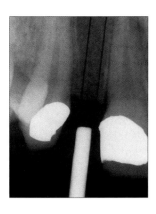

Fig 9   Periapical radiograph showing the radiographic rod, highlighting the proposed implant mesiodistal angulation.

A periapical radiograph was taken with the template in place to confirm the planned implant position, avoiding the adjacent tooth roots (Fig 9). The surgical template was then fabricated based upon the confirmed radiographic pin position (Fig 10).

At the surgical visit, a scalloping procedure using the vacuform (vertical) template was performed to allow proper vertical placement of the NN implant. The surgical template and drill sleeve was used to prepare the osteotomy site (Fig 11).

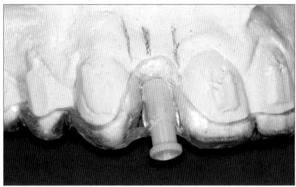

Fig 10   Diagnostic cast with surgical template and drill sleeve in place.

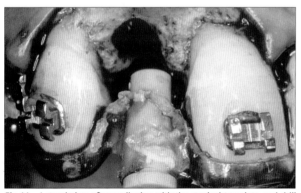

Fig 11   Lateral view after scalloping with the surgical template and drill sleeve in place before the preparation of osteotomy site.

Once the implant had been placed, the vertical depth (shoulder 2 mm apically of the proposed mucosal margin) was confirmed before the transfer part was removed. After the placement of the healing cap and suturing, a periapical radiograph was taken (Figs 12a-c). The pontic on the orthodontic wire was adjusted so that the healing cap was out of contact. The patient was scheduled for a follow-up visit after one week.

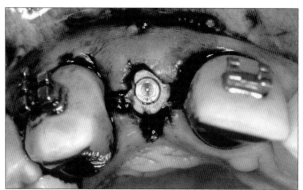

Fig 12a   Occlusal view of the healing cap.

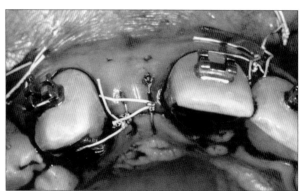

Fig 12b   Occlusal view after suturing.

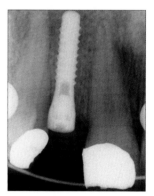

Fig 12c   Postoperative radiograph.

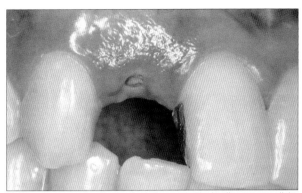

Fig 13   Twelve weeks after implant placement. The healing cap was slightly exposed, allowing access to the implant shoulder without the need for tissue removal.

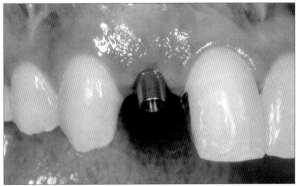

Fig 14a   Lateral view with an unprepared titanium coping in place. Indicator grooves were made mid-facially and in any areas requiring reduction for interocclusal and interarch space.

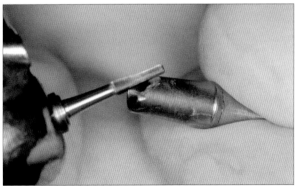

Fig 14b   Extraoral preparation of the titanium coping with a high-speed carbide bur.

Twelve weeks after implant placement, the patient was scheduled for a loading visit (Fig 13). Loading of the NN implant occurred at twelve weeks because it had a titanium-plasma sprayed surface (TPS); all NN implants today have a sandblasted large-grit acid-etched (SLA) surface that allows loading after six weeks of healing.

At this appointment, a provisional restoration was made that would initiate the maturation of the transition zone. After the removal of the healing cap, a titanium coping was hand-tightened, and indicator grooves were prepared on the surface with a high-speed carbide bur that would assist in an appropriate reduction extraorally (Figs 14a, b).

Once the custom preparation was complete, the coping was placed onto the implant and hand-tightened and the access hole was blocked with cotton before the provisional restoration was fabricated (Fig 15).

A vacuform retainer of the waxup was used with methylmethacrylate resin to fabricate the provisional restoration. Once the provisional material had set intraorally, it was removed along with the coping and placed back onto a laboratory analog (Fig 16). Methyl methacrylate powder and monomer was mixed in a dappen dish and added to the provisional with a brush to create an emergence profile from the coping margin to the contact point, establishing support for the transition zone (Fig 17).

After the emergence modifications of the provisional were complete, the coping was returned to the implant and tightened to 15 Ncm and covered with cotton pellets, and the provisional was seated. Blanching of the tissue subsided within 10 minutes, so that the provisional was cemented with a temporary cement (Fig 18). The occlusion was adjusted and the patient was scheduled to return to the clinic for a final impression after four weeks.

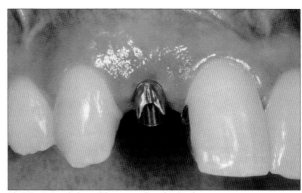

Fig 15   Lateral view with prepared coping in place.

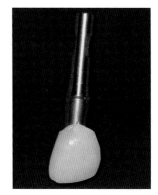

Fig 16   The provisional restoration on the coping and laboratory analog. Peri-implant tissue prevented the acrylic resin from extending submucosally, creating an overhang between the acrylic resin and the coping.

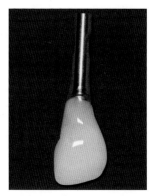

Fig 17   Acrylic resin was added to create an emergence profile to support the interproximal tissue and create a facial soft-tissue margin.

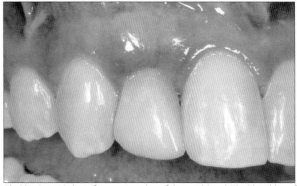

Fig 18   Lateral view after cementation of the provisional. The blanching of the tissue had subsided.

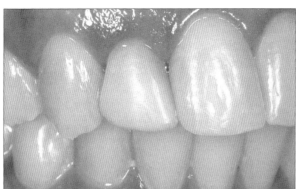

Fig 19   Lateral view four weeks after insertion of the provisional restoration.

The patient returned after four weeks for a final impression. The tissue had begun the maturation process, and the mucosal margin looked more refined (Fig 19).

Before the final impression, a periapical radiograph was taken and the correct shade determined (Figs 20a, b).

Upon removal of the provisional restoration, the matured transition zone was exposed (Fig 21).

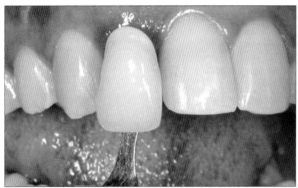

Fig 20a   The selected shade tab in place.

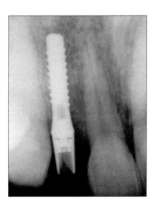

Fig 20b   Periapical radiograph with the titanium coping and provisional restoration in place.

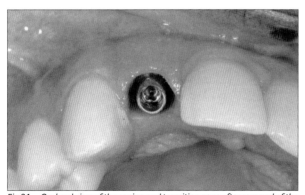

Fig 21   Occlusal view of the coping and transition zone after removal of the provisional restoration.

The tissue scallop created by the provisional was larger than the diameter of the impression cap. To prevent the collapse of this tissue as the impression was taken, a custom impression cap was fabricated extraorally from the provisional restoration (Figs 22a-c).

Once modified, the impression cap was placed on the implant shoulder, and a polyvinyl siloxane impression was made (Fig 23).

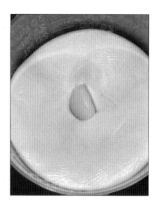

Fig 22a Fabricating a custom impression cap. The provisional on the titanium coping and analog are embedded in silicone putty.

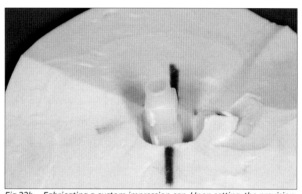

Fig 22b Fabricating a custom impression cap. Upon setting, the provisional and coping were carefully removed and an impression cap was snapped onto the analog. Orofacial indicators were marked into the putty to retain the orientation of the cap for placement in the mouth. A pattern resin material (GC Resin, GC America) was flowed into the void that existed around the cap and allowed to set.

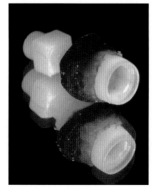

Fig 22c Fabricating a custom impression cap. The modified impression cap upon removal from the putty matrix. The pattern resin has captured the transition zone.

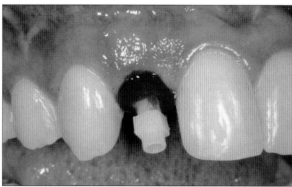

Fig 23 Customized NN snap-on impression cap in place before taking the final impression.

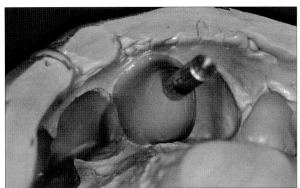

Fig 24   A polysulfide material was placed around the analog and custom impression cap.

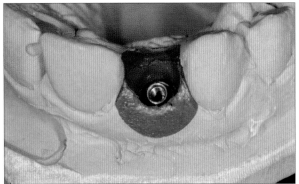

Fig 25   An occlusal view of the master cast with the soft-tissue analog highlighting the transition zone.

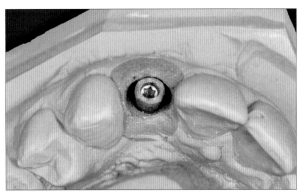

Fig 26   After reduction of the oxidizable NN framework blank and before application of ceramic.

Once set, the final impression was removed from the mouth, and a laboratory analog was placed into the impression cap. A polysulfide material was injected around the analog area and allowed to set (Fig 24).

A low-expansion die stone was then poured into the final impression and allowed to set. The transition zone was visible on the master cast after the impression had been removed (Fig 25).

The NN framework blank (oxidizable) was chosen by the laboratory as the definitive coping. This blank allowed the technician to build up ceramic on its surface and created support for the peri-implant tissue while generating a cement line closer to the soft-tissue margin. Traditionally, these custom abutments are made with a gold alloy; more recently, CAD/CAM technology and titanium have increasingly been used. Due to the patient's esthetic expectations, it was decided to place ceramic material under the tissue surface, preventing any submucosal reflection of the metal. Once the framework blank had been placed onto the master cast, it was reduced to provide space for the ceramic material (Fig 26).

An opaque was then applied, followed by a buildup designed to support the soft-tissue analog and maintain a submucosal margin position (Fig 27).

Upon completion of the customized abutment, a ceramo-metal crown was fabricated with a 360° ceramic butt-joint margin (Fig 28).

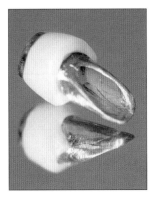

Fig 27   Customized framework blank. Emergence profile in ceramic instead of the traditional gold alloy.

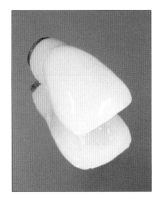

Fig 28   The customized framework blank and ceramo-metal crown ready for insertion.

At the insertion visit three weeks after the final impression session, the provisional restoration and framework blank were removed (Fig 29).

The implant was irrigated with the air-water syringe before the customized blank was inserted. Once the fit and shade of the final restoration had been confirmed, the screw was tightened to 35 Ncm (Figs 30a, b).

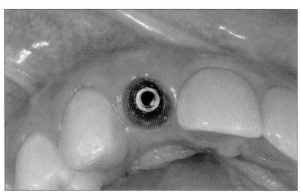

Fig 29   Occlusal view of the implant shoulder before placement of the customized framework blank.

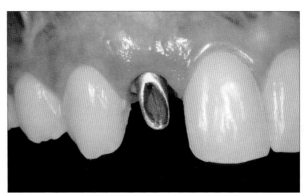

Fig 30a   Lateral view of the customized framework blank in place before crown cementation.

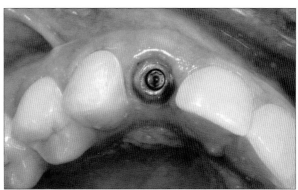

Fig 30b   Occlusal view of the customized framework blank in place before crown cementation. The ceramic margin is located slightly below the mucosa, thus allowing for easy post-cementation access.

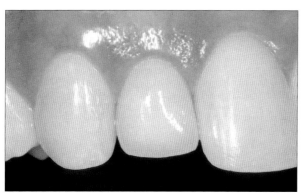

Fig 31a   Lateral view of the inserted implant-supported crown on tooth 12.

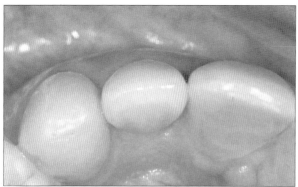

Fig 31b   Occlusal view of the inserted implant-supported crown on tooth 12.

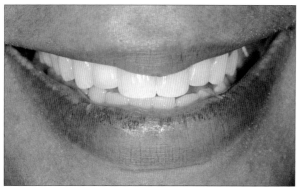

Fig 31c   Post-treatment smile.

The screw access hole was covered with a cotton pellet and sealed with Cavit (3M Espe). The final restoration was cemented with permanent cement, and the occlusion was adjusted to a light shim-stock pull (Figs 31a-c). Adjustments to the ceramic surface were followed by a polishing procedure with diamond-impregnated disks that helped create a glaze-like ceramic surface.

A periapical radiograph was taken and the patient was scheduled for follow-up after three weeks (Fig 32). At the three-week visit, the peri-implant tissues were examined for cement residue, and the occlusion was checked. Oral hygiene and home-care procedures were reviewed with the patient. At the end of the visit, the patient was scheduled for yearly maintenance.

The patient was seen after her maintenance visit for a follow-up at four years (Figs 33a, b).

Acknowledgments

Orthodontic Procedures
Department of Orthodontics, Baylor College of Dentistry, Dallas, Texas, USA

Surgical Procedures
Dr. Farhad Boltchi – Private Practice, Arlington, Texas, USA

Laboratory Procedures
Eloy Henry – Dallas, Texas, USA

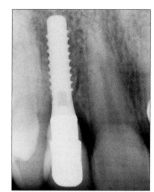

Fig 32   Periapical radiograph of the implant-supported crown on tooth 12.

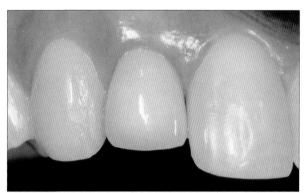

Fig 33a   Lateral view of the implant-supported crown on tooth 12, four years after insertion.

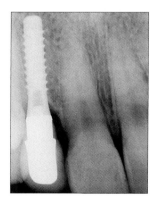

Fig 33b   Periapical radiograph of the implant-supported crown on tooth 12, four years after insertion.

5 Esthetic Complications and Their Causes

D. Buser, W. C. Martin

5.1 Introduction

Esthetic complications with implant-supported restorations can be either iatrogenic or caused by anatomic factors such as bone or soft-tissue deficiencies. In many patients with esthetic complications, a combination of several factors is present. A thorough understanding of these factors is therefore important to be able to improve esthetic treatment outcomes in daily practice.

Iatrogenic causes of esthetic complications include:
• Selection of an inappropriate, oversized implant (wide platform)
• Malpositioned implant entering a danger zone in a coronoapical, mesiodistal or orofacial direction
• A surgical approach that overstresses the healing capacity of the tissues, leading to the resorption of the facial bone wall
• Improper use or non-use of provisional restorations to shape the peri-implant soft tissues
• Inappropriate use of restorative implant components or materials for fabricating restorations

Anatomic causes of esthetic complications include:
• Horizontal or vertical bone deficiencies at the implant site
• Vertical bone deficiencies at adjacent root surfaces
• Implant sites with multiple missing teeth leading to the placement of adjacent implants

For single-tooth replacement, the factor of adjacent implants plays no role and will not be discussed in this Treatment Guide. A separate Treatment Guide will be devoted to this issue.

These factors will be discussed with seven reports on cases with esthetic complications. Each case will be systematically analyzed to improve the reader's understanding of these problems.

5.2 Case Reports

5.2.1 Patient No. 1

A 20-year-old female patient presented with a compromised esthetic treatment outcome after implant therapy in the anterior maxilla. Figure 1 shows the clinical status 4 months after implant restoration in the area of the right central incisor. The patient presented with a high lip-line situation exposing not only the crowns, but also the gingiva when smiling.

The close-up view shows the full extent of the interruption of the harmonious gingival line by a soft-tissue recession at the implant-supported crown (Fig 2). The gingival recession measures approximately 3 mm and developed rapidly within a few weeks after the insertion of the implant crown.

The periapical radiograph reveals the cause for the esthetic failure (Fig 3): The implant shoulder was placed too far apically using an extensive countersinking procedure. In addition, the implant was also malpositioned in a mesiodistal direction, since the implant shoulder almost touched the root surface of the lateral incisor. Both these factors led to bone resorption on the facial aspect of the implant and on the adjacent root surface of the lateral incisor.

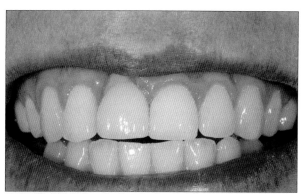

Fig 1   The high lip-line situation clearly reveals the interruption of the harmonious gingival line.

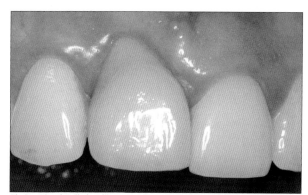

Fig 2   The detail view illustrates the extent of the gingival recession at the implant crown.

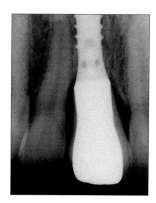

Fig 3   Periapical radiograph showing the malposition of the implant in a coronoapical and in a mesiodistal direction.

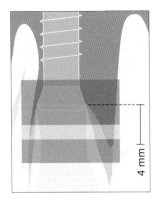

Fig 4   The implant in apical malposition due to excessive countersinking and the close proximity of the implant to the lateral incisor.

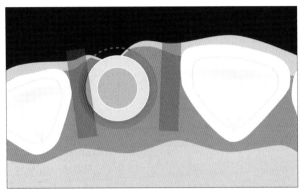

Fig 5   The "bone saucer" (red) causes facial bone wall resorption if the facial bone wall is only 1 mm in thickness.

Figure 4 illustrates the coronoapical implant position in relation to the correct coronoapical implant position for this case. The implant shoulder is located approximately 4 mm apical to the cemento-enamel junction (CEJ) of the adjacent central incisor. The correct distance to the CEJ should only be 1 mm.

The peri-implant "bone saucer" that routinely forms around dental implants after prosthetic restoration can lead to a partial resorption of the facial bone wall and subsequent facial soft-tissue recession when the implant is placed in the apical danger zone, since it has a vertical extension of about 1.5 to 2.0 mm and a horizontal component of 1.0 to 1.5 mm (Buser and coworkers, 2004) (Fig 5).

When the peri-implant "bone saucer" had developed around this particular implant after loading, it added to the resorption of the facial bone wall. As a result, facial soft-tissue recession rapidly developed within a few weeks. The graphic also shows a malposition of the implant shoulder in the mesiodistal danger zone of the adjacent lateral incisor.

Case summary:
The soft-tissue recession of 3 mm was mainly caused by a malposition of the implant shoulder in the coronoapical direction. The complication cannot be resolved by mucogingival surgery. Due to the high lip-line situation of the patient, the only option to resolve the recession is to remove the implant. From a surgical point of view, this is very difficult due to the close proximity of the implant to the lateral incisor. The removal of the implant will not only create a bone defect at the implant site, but also a shortened mesial papilla at the lateral incisor.

5.2.2 Patient No. 2

This 40-year-old female patient was referred with a serious esthetic complication. She presented with a major gingival recession at the implant crown in the area of tooth 12. The main cause of this complication was a severe implant malposition in coronoapical direction. The implant shoulder was positioned about 5 mm apical to the planned soft-tissue margin of the future implant-supported crown. This malposition resulted in severe facial bone resorption and subsequent soft-tissue recession. The use of pink ceramic was necessary to mask the unfavorable esthetic treatment outcome (Fig 6).

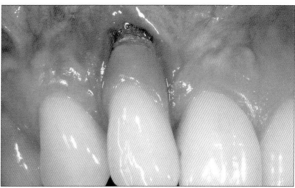

Fig 6   Severe esthetic complication with the implant crown at site 12.

The periapical radiograph reveals the apical malposition of the implant that caused the severe esthetic complication (Fig 7).

The patient exhibited a mid lip-line situation. When she was smiling, the severe soft-tissue recession was partially covered by the lip (Fig 8).

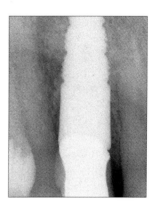

Fig 7   Periapical radiograph demonstrating a well-integrated implant in an apical malposition.

Case summary:
The severe soft-tissue recession was mainly caused by an extreme apical malposition of the implant shoulder. Due to the mid lip-line situation, the esthetic complication was marginally acceptable to the patient.

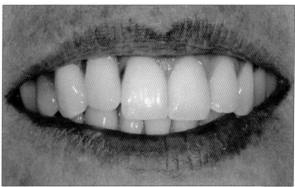

Fig 8   The patient's mid lip-line situation masking the compromised treatment outcome.

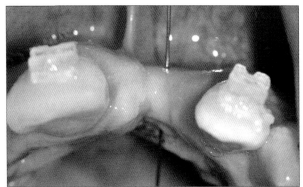

Fig 9   An attempt to "sound" for osseous support revealed a deficiency in vertical and horizontal bone

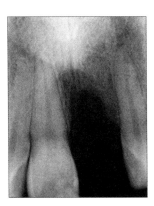

Fig 10   Periapical radiograph confirming bone deficiencies at the proposed implant site and interproximal support on the adjacent roots.

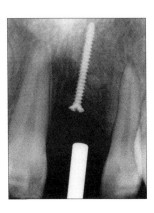

Fig 11   Periapical radiograph with the radiographic template in place.

5.2.3   Patient No. 3

A 30-year-old female patient presented at the clinic for a consultation to replace a missing tooth (21) lost in a sport accident. Examination of the esthetic risk for her treatment revealed a medium lip line at full smile, exposing three-quarters of the clinical crowns and the tips of the papillae. The gingival biotype was thin, with highly scalloped papillae, tapered clinical crowns, and a thin band of keratinized tissue. The site analysis showed a deficiency in osseous width and height extending apically of the middle third of the adjacent roots (Fig 9).

The periapical radiograph confirmed this bone loss while showing that adequate bone support existed on the interproximal of the adjacent teeth 11 and 22 (Fig 10).

Based upon the clinical findings, the patient was informed of the high risk of esthetic failure with dental implant therapy. A plan was presented to address the hard-tissue and soft-tissue deficiencies prior to implant placement. Six months after the grafting procedure, a clinical examination revealed successful horizontal bone regeneration, while a deficiency in vertical height remained. The patient declined further tissue-enhancement procedures and desired to proceed with implant placement. A radiographic template was fabricated and a periapical radiograph taken (Fig 11).

The dental implant was placed within the orofacial and mesiodistal comfort zones, while entering the coronoapical danger zone (Fig 12).

Six weeks later, the implant was restored with a provisional restoration; the clinical result highlighted the apical position of the soft-tissue margin at site 21 related to the adjacent teeth (Fig 13).

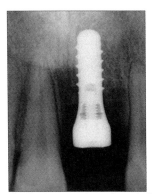

Fig 12   Postoperative radiograph depicting the placement of the implant in the coronoapical danger zone.

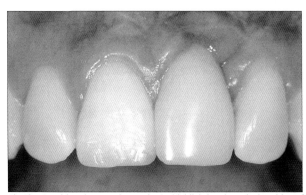

Fig 13   Provisional restoration at site 21 highlighting the apical position of the soft-tissue margin related to the adjacent teeth.

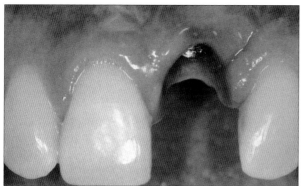

Fig 14   Clinical view of implant 21 highlighting the apical position of the soft-tissue margin relative to the adjacent teeth. The interproximal tissue support was promising.

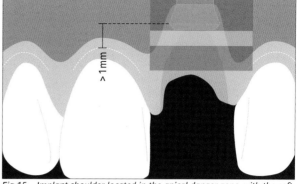

Fig 15   Implant shoulder located in the apical danger zone, with the soft-tissue margin in an apical position.

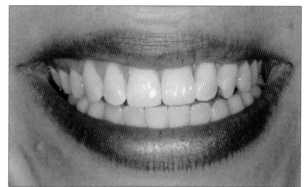

Fig 16   At full smile, the facial tissue deficiency was not visible.

Upon maturation of the transition zone, there was interproximal tissue support, but a mucosal deficiency on the facial aspect was evident (Fig 14).

The implant shoulder was located in the apical danger zone (Fig 15). To compensate for this situation, pink ceramic material was integrated into the implant-supported superstructure. In this way, a pleasing esthetic treatment outcome could be achieved despite the compromised clinical situation (Fig 16).

The esthetic result was acceptable to the patient (Fig 17).

The postoperative periapical radiograph highlights the final position of the supporting structures (Fig 18).

Case summary:
This clinical case is an example of an esthetic compromise associated with clinician and patient causes and anatomical limitations. The challenges in this treatment were associated with several factors: patient limitations—time constraints and finances; surgical challenges—extensive grafting procedures with multiple procedure limits; and anatomic limitations—thin biotype coupled with severe localized atrophy. Proper esthetic risk assessment, patient education, treatment planning, and technician expertise allowed a pleasing esthetic treatment outcome, since the necessary compromises were take into consideration before the treatment began.

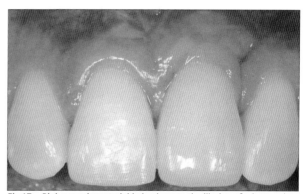

Fig 17   Pink ceramic material helped create the illusion of a harmonious soft-tissue contour.

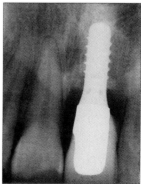

Fig 18   Periapical radiograph after insertion highlighting the final positions of the dental implant and surrounding hard tissues.

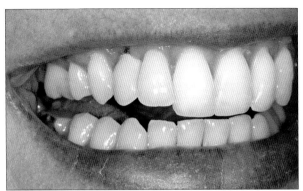

Fig 19   The high lip line exposes the metal margin of the implant crown when smiling.

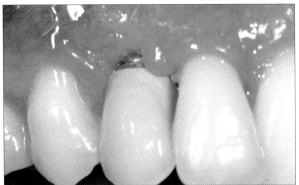

Fig 20   Detail view of the esthetic complication. The metal margin was visible and the mesial papilla was clearly shortened.

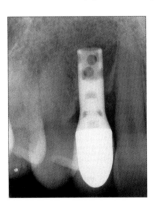

Fig 21   The periapical radiograph reveals the oversized implant that resulted in the implant shoulder being located in the mesial danger zone. As a result, the bone between the implant and the adjacent lateral incisor was resorbed, leading to the reduction of the mesial papilla.

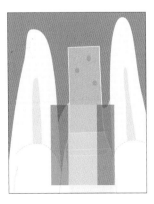

Fig 22 The implant invades the mesial danger zone, leading to the resorption of alveolar bone at the adjacent lateral incisor.

5.2.4   Patient No. 4

This 34-year-old female patient presented with an unsatisfactory esthetic treatment outcome, a visible implant shoulder at tooth 13 and a reduced papilla mesially of the implant-supported superstructure (Fig 19). The patient had a high lip-line situation, so that the metal margin of the implant crown was in plain view when she smiled.

The papilla mesial to the implant crown was reduced, and the metal margins of the implant shoulder and of the ceramo-metal crown were visible (Fig 20). Both complications have clear causes. The visible metal margin had been caused by a malposition in the coronoapical direction; this implant shoulder was positioned in the coronal danger zone. That the implant was not placed sufficiently deeply into the tissue. In addition, the concavity on the facial aspect gave rise to the assumption that the facial bone wall was lacking in support for the facial soft tissue.

The periapical radiograph showed the cause for the short mesial papilla of the implant crown. The diameter of the implant selected for this single-tooth gap was too large, so the Regular Neck implant had entered the mesial danger zone of the adjacent lateral incisor. This close proximity led to alveolar bone resorption between the implant and root surfaces, followed by the shrinkage of the papilla. To avoid this unpleasant complication, orthodontic treatment would have been required to open the mesiodistal space in this single-tooth gap, allowing for an appropriate placement of a Regular Neck implant. The use of a Narrow Neck implant to replace an upper canine is contraindicated.

Figure 22 shows the actual implant position in relation to the comfort and danger zones in the mesiodistal direction.

Case summary:
The esthetic complication observed has two causes – first, the inappropriate, oversized implant that made the implant shoulder invade the mesial danger zone at the adjacent lateral incisor, causing bone resorption there and subsequently a short mesial papilla. Secondly, the coronoapical malposition led to an exposed metal margin. To resolve this, the preparation of the implant shoulder on the facial and mesial aspect and the fabrication of a new crown can help improve the esthetic outcome without the removal of the implant.

5.2.5 Patient No. 5

This 43-year-old female patient presented with an esthetic disaster. She had been treated with an immediate implant following extraction of tooth 21. The patient had a high lip-line that exposed the facial soft tissue when she smiled (Fig 23).

Following implant placement, a severe soft-tissue recession developed within a few months, exposing a significant portion of the implant surface (Fig 24). On the day of examination, the implant showed slight mobility and had to be removed.

The implant shoulder was located too far facially, drastically invading the facial danger zone (Figs 25, 26). This is partly due to the selection of an oversized implant. Such an implant position can be also caused by the anatomy of the alveolus in immediate implants, since the alveolus guides the drills too far facially.

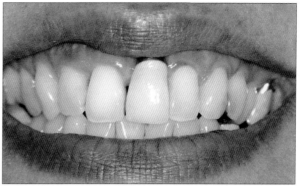

Fig 23   The patient's high lip line exposed the esthetic failure when she smiled.

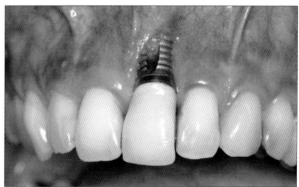

Fig 24   Close-up view showing the extent of the soft-tissue recession.

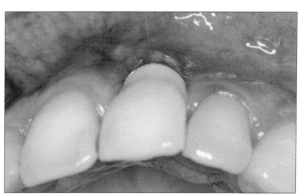

Fig 25   Occlusal view revealing the facial malposition of the implant.

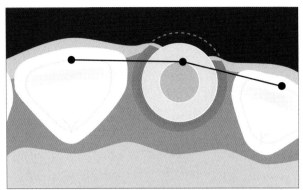

Fig 26 The oversized implant was malpositioned and entered the facial danger zone. The facial bone wall had been completely resorbed during the healing period despite an attempt to build up the facial bone wall with a simultaneous GBR procedure.

The periapical radiograph illustrated the oversized implant in the area of the central incisor (Fig 27). The use of a wide-platform implant aggravated the effect of the malposition.

Case summary:
- This esthetic disaster had been caused by (a) the inappropriate selection of a wide platform implant and (b) an inappropriate treatment approach using the concept of immediate implant placement following extraction. This approach led to a malposition and invasion of the facial danger zone. In addition, the simultaneous GBR procedure could not regenerate a facial bone wall of sufficient height and thickness due to the malposition of the wide-diameter implant.
- The removal of the implant was the only solution to eliminate the esthetic failure. However, this implant removal created a severe bone and soft-tissue defect in the alveolar crest that is difficult to handle given all the forensic problems involved in such a treatment.

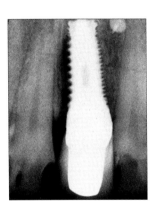

Fig 27 The implant is clearly too large in relation to the gap size, resulting in bone resorption.

5.2.6 Patient No. 6

A 70-year-old female patient presented at the clinic for placement of an implant at site 22. Six months previously the site had been augmented with an allogenous graft (Fig 28). An implant was placed without the use of a surgical template. A surgical index was created at the time of surgery to assist in the second-stage provisional fabrication.

The postoperative periapical radiograph revealed that the implant had been placed in the apical danger zone (Fig 29).

In the laboratory, the surgical index was used to confirm the position of the dental implant (Figs 30a, b).

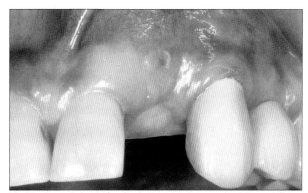

Fig 28   Frontal view before implant surgery. Interproximal tissue deficiencies are evident adjacent to site 22.

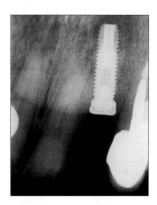

Fig 29   Postoperative periapical radiograph highlighting the "deep" placement of the dental implant compared to the adjacent teeth. Deficiencies in interproximal bone support were evident on the teeth adjacent to site 22.

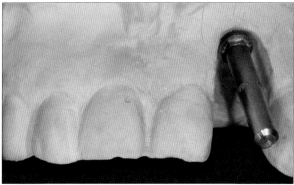

Fig 30a   Master cast highlighting the extreme facial and apical position of the implant.

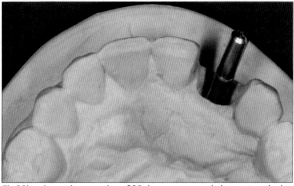

Fig 30b   An angle correction of 25 degrees was needed to restore the implant.

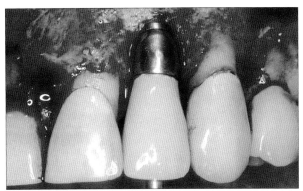

Fig 31   A 25-degree abutment and a screw-retained restoration were delivered during second-stage surgery.

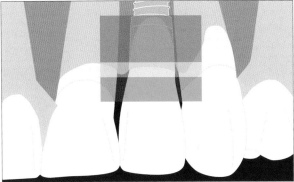

Fig 32   The apical placement of the implant caused bone recession and subsequently also soft-tissue recession.

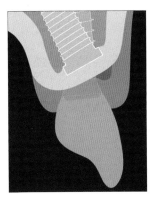

Fig 33   The invasion of the facial danger zone aggravated the resorption process.

It was decided to fabricate a definitive screw-retained restoration for insertion during second-stage surgery (Fig 31).

The implant was clearly placed too far apically (Fig 32) and too far facially (Fig 33).

During second-stage surgery, an attempt to increase the soft-tissue support was made using a subepithelial connective-tissue graft (Fig 34).

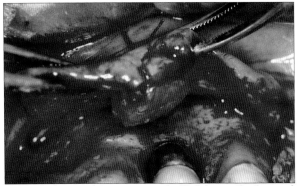

Fig 34   During second-stage surgery, a subepithelial connective-tissue graft was used in an attempt to increase the soft-tissue volume.

The clinical result immediately after surgery was favorable (Fig 35).

At the one-year follow-up visit, interproximal and facial tissue loss was evident due to a lack of interproximal and facial bone support (Fig 36).

The periapical radiograph revealed the loss of peri-implant support as well as the unfavorable crown-to-implant ratio (Fig 37).

Case summary:
This esthetic and functional compromise was necessitated by the incorrect application of the planning principles for ideal implant placement. The clinical disregard for comfort and danger zones during surgery led to an implant position that was restoratively and functionally difficult to manage. Any attempt to overcome the lack of osseous support after implant placement inevitably had to meet with failure.

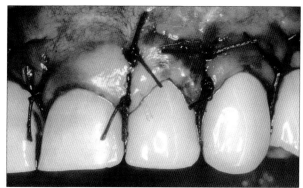
Fig 35   Postoperative frontal view showing an acceptable result.

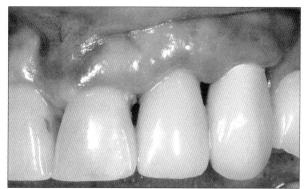
Fig 36   One-year follow-up revealing the side effects of inadequate peri-implant hard-tissue support.

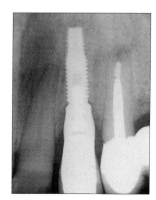
Fig 37   Periapical radiograph at one-year follow-up. Poor implant-to-crown ratio.

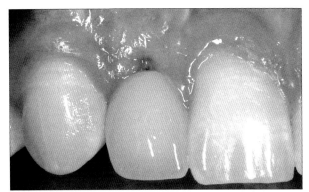

Fig 38   Lateral view at site 12 with titanium visible at the soft-tissue margin.

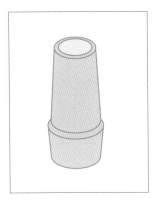

Fig 39   Narrow Neck titanium coping.

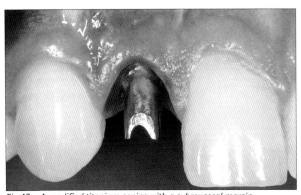

Fig 40   A modified titanium coping with a submucosal margin.

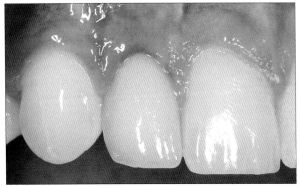

Fig 41   A pleasing esthetic result with a properly restored implant at site 12.

5.2.7   Patient No. 7

A 23-year-old female patient presented at the clinic with an esthetic compromise of an implant-supported restoration at tooth 12. The patient reported an unsatisfactory restorative result with titanium visible at the mucosal margin (Fig 38).

A clinical examination revealed a submucosal implant shoulder. Research on the implant system (Narrow Neck implant) and restorative components (titanium coping) showed an error in the use of the implant components. The titanium coping was a modifiable coping, allowing the restorative margin to be placed in a submucosal position (Fig 39).

The correction necessitated the removal of the crown and coping. A new customized coping and a ceramo-metal crown were fabricated (Fig 40).

An esthetically pleasing result was obtained (Fig 41). A periapical radiograph was taken to confirm full seating of the restoration (Fig 42).

Case summary:
This esthetic compromise had been caused by an inappropriate choice of components for the implant system used. Although the implant was ideally placed in all comfort zones, the improper use of the titanium coping resulted in an unesthetic appearance. The correction was easy to accomplish, requiring only the proper preparation of a new coping and crown. The result was an acceptable esthetic implant restoration.

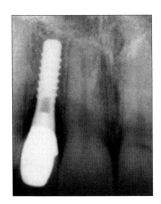

Fig 42   Periapical radiograph taken after insertion of the definitive restoration.

5.3 Conclusions

These seven case reports demonstrate several possible causes of esthetic implant complications or implant failures. In the majority of such cases, an inappropriate implant selection using wide-platform implants, an inappropriate implant position invading one or several danger zones, or the use of an inappropriate treatment approach that overstresses the biologic healing capacity of the peri-implant hard and soft tissues causes these complications.

These iatrogenic factors are often combined with anatomic risk factors such as horizontal or vertical bone deficiencies.

These esthetic implant complications or failures often require the removal of the implant, leading to bone or soft-tissue deficiencies.

6 <u>Synopsis</u>

U. C. Belser

The main objectives of this volume of the ITI Treatment Guide were to comprehensively address the therapeutic situation "single-tooth restoration in the anterior maxilla" and to provide the clinician with relevant information and state-of-the-art knowledge on both surgical and prosthetic procedures. Primary importance was given to predictable, evidence-based concepts and derived practical procedures, specifically encompassing the following aspects:

- Treatment goals, including the patient's demands and expectations.
- Preoperative diagnostics.
- Case-specific esthetic risk assessment and determination of individual complexity level.
- Definitions and guidelines for achieving a satisfactory three-dimensional implant position.
- Prosthetic management, including an overview of the various restorative options and the associated decision-making criteria, as well as precise guidelines related to the recommended clinical and laboratory step-by-step procedures.
- Analysis of possible causes of complications.

Special emphasis was put on the systematic assessment of the individual esthetic risk of a given patient. This comprised the identification and weighing of both general and local risk factors. The focus was on clinical cases with a risk profile compatible with implant therapy. In this context, assessment of the individual complexity of the initial situation should also provide the relevant information to the clinician as to whether the collaboration of a surgical specialist should be considered.

Furthermore, the direct association between the complexity of the case and the importance of adhering to scientifically proven protocols was pointed out specifically.

Similarly, for the prosthetic phase of therapy, the application of sound, evidence-based clinical and laboratory protocols was underlined as being of the utmost importance. In particular, it was pointed out that sufficient time must be given to developing healthy, stable, and esthetic peri-implant soft-tissue conditions.

The proposed decision trees for Regular Neck (RN) and Narrow Neck (NN) implants were developed to facilitate the respective decision-making processes for the specific design of the provisional and restorative components of the final superstructure including the selection of the respective restorative components. These decisions depended mainly on the individual implant position, which included both implantation depth and implant axis.

A comprehensive series of cases were presented to exemplify the consensus statements and to recommend specific prosthetic approaches, optimally adapted to the individual situation of each patient.

Finally, a number of clinical examples of complications and failures were used to identify a variety of possible causes of esthetic shortcomings and to make recommendations for their prevention.

7 <u>Literature/References</u>

Abrahamsson I, Berglundh T, Glanz PO, Lindhe J. The mucosal attachment at different abutments. An experimental study in dogs. J Clin Periodontol. 1998 Sep;25(9):721 – 7.

Andersson B, Taylor A, Lang BR, Scheller H, Scharer P, Sorensen JA, Tarnow D. Alumina ceramic implant abutments used for single-tooth replacement: a prospective 1- to 3-year multicenter study. Int J Prosthodont. 2001 Sep-Oct;14:432 – 38.

Alpert A. A rationale for attached gingiva at the soft-tissue/implant interface: esthetic and functional dictates. Compendium. 1994 Mar;15(3):356, 358, 360 – 2 passim; quiz 368.

Bain CA, Moy PK. The association between the failure of dental implants and cigarette smoking. Int J Oral Maxillofac Impl. 1993;8;609 – 15.

Belser U, Bernard JP, Buser D. Implant-supported restorations in the anterior region: Prosthetic considerations. Pract Periodontics Aesthet Dent. 1996 Nov-Dec; 8(9):857 – 83; quiz 884.

Belser U, Buser D, Hess D, Schmid B, Bernard JP, Lang K. Aesthetic implant restorations in partially edentulous patients: A critical appraisal. Periodontol. 2000. 1998 Jun;17:132 – 50.

Belser UC, Bernard JP, Buser D. Implant placement in the esthetic zone. In: Lindhe J, Karring T, Lang NP, editors. Clinical Periodontology and Implant Dentistry, 4th ed. Blackwell Munksgaard; 2003:915 – 44.

Belser U, Buser D, Higginbottom F. Consensus statements and recommended clinical procedures regarding esthetics in implant dentistry. Int J Oral Maxillofac Implants. 2004;19 Suppl:73 – 4.

Belser U, Schmid B, Higginbottom F, Buser D. Outcome analysis of implant restorations located in the anterior maxilla: a review of the recent literature. Int J Oral Maxillofac Implants. 2004;19 Suppl: 30 – 42.

Bernard JP, Schatz JP, Christou P, Belser U, Kiliaridis S.: Long-term vertical changes of anterior maxillary teeth adjacent to single implants in young and mature adults. A retrospective study. J Clin Periodontol. 2004 Nov;31(11):1024 – 8.

Botticelli D, Berglundh T, Lindhe J: Hard-tissue alterations following immediate implant placement in extraction sockets. J Clin Periodontol. 2004;31(10),820 – 8.

Buser D, Dahlin C, Schenk RK, editors. Guided bone regeneration in implant dentistry. Chicago: Quintessence; 1994.

Buser D, von Arx T. Surgical procedures in partially edentulous patients with ITI implants. Clin Oral Implants Res. 2000;11 Suppl. 1:83 – 100.

Buser D, Martin W, Belser U. Optimizing esthetics for implant restorations in the anterior maxilla: anatomic and surgical considerations. Int J Oral Maxillofac Implants. 2004;19 Suppl:43 – 61.

Cardaropoli D, Re S, Corrente G, Abundo R. Reconstruction of the maxillary midline papilla following a combined orthodontic-periodontic treatment in adult periodontal patients. J Clin Periodontol. 2004 Feb;31(2):79 – 84.

Choquet V, Hermans M, Adriaenssens P, Daelemans P, Tarnow DP, Malevez C. Clinical and radiographic evaluation of the papilla level adjacent to single-tooth dental implants. A retrospective study in the maxillary anterior region. J Periodontol. 2001 Oct;72(10):1364 – 71.

De Bruyn H, Collaert B. The effect of smoking on early implant failure. Clin Oral Implants Res. 1994 Dec;5(4):260 – 4.

Ekfeldt A, Eriksson A, Johansson LA. Peri-implant mucosal level in patients treated with implant-supported fixed prostheses: a 1-year follow-up study. Int J Prosthodont. 2003 Sep-Oct;16(5):529 – 32.

Ellegaard B, Baelum V, Karring T. Implant therapy in periodontally compromised patients. Clin Oral Implants Res. 1997 Jun;8(3):180 – 8.

Esposito M, Ekkestube A, Gröndahl K. Radiological evaluation of marginal bone loss at tooth surfaces facing single Brånemark implants. Clin Oral Implants Res. 1993 Sep;4(3):151 – 7.

Feloutzis A, Lang NP, Tonetti MS, Burgin W, Bragger U, Buser D, et al. IL-1 gene polymorphism and smoking as risk factors for peri-implant bone loss in a well-maintained population. Clin Oral Implants Res. 2003 Feb;14(1):10 – 7.

Francetti L, Trombelli L, Lombardo G, Guida L, Cafiero C, Roccuzzo M, et al. Evaluation of efficacy of enamel matrix derivative in the treatment of intrabony defects: a 24-month multicenter study. Int J Periodontics Restorative Dent. 2005 Oct;25(5):461 – 73.

Garber DA, Belser UC. Restoration-driven implant placement with restoration-driven site development. Compend Contin Educ Dent. 1995 Aug;16(8):796–804.

Giannopoulou C, Bernard JP, Buser D, Carrel A, Belser UC. Effect of intracrevicular restoration margins on peri-implant health: clinical, biochemical, and microbiologic findings around esthetic implants up to 9 years. Int J of Oral Maxillofac Implants. 2003 Mar-Apr;18(2):173–81.

Gruica B, Wang HY, Lang NP, Buser D. Impact of IL-1 genotype and smoking status on the prognosis of osseointegrated implants. Clin Oral Implants Res. 2004 Aug;15(4):393–400.

Grunder U. Stability of the mucosal topography around single-tooth implants and adjacent teeth: 1-year results. Int J Periodontics Restorative Dent. 2000 Feb; 20 (1):11–7.

Hämmerle CH, Jung RE. Bone augmentation by means of barrier membranes. Periodontol. 2000. 2003;33:36–53.

Hämmerle C, Glauser R, Jung R, Pjetursson B, Ramel C. Orale Implantologie: Aktuelle Schwerpunkte für die Klinik. ("Oral Implantology: Current Clinical Focus."): Zurich: Clinic for Dental Crown and Bridge Prosthetics, Partial Prosthetics, and Dental Material Science, Center for Dental and Oral Medicine and Cranio-Maxillofacial Surgery, University of Zurich. 2005;129–49.

Hämmerle CHF, Chen ST, Wilson TG Jr: Consensus statements and recommended clinical procedures regarding the placement of implants in extraction sockets. Int J Oral Maxillofac Implants. 2004;19 Suppl:26–8.

Hermann JS, Buser D. Guided bone regeneration for dental implants. Curr Opin Periodontol. 1996;3:168–77.

Hermann JS, Cochran DL, Nummikoski PV, Buser D. Crestal bone changes around titanium implants. A radiographic evaluation of unloaded nonsubmerged and submerged implants in the canine mandible. J Periodontol. 1997 Nov;68(11): 1117–30.

Hermann JS, Buser D, Schenk RK, Cochran DL. Crestal bone changes around titanium implants. A histometric evaluation of unloaded nonsubmerged and submerged implants in the canine mandible. J Periodontol. 2000 Sep;71(9):1412–24.

Higginbottom FL, Wilson TG Jr. Three-dimensional templates for placement of root-form dental implants: a technical note. Int J Oral Maxillofac Implants. 1996 Nov-Dec; 11(6):787–93.

Higginbottom F, Belser U, Jones J, Keith S. Prosthetic management of implants in the esthetic zone. Int J Oral Maxillofac Implants. 2004;19 Suppl.:62–72.

Hinds KF: Custom impression coping for an exact registration of the healed tissue in the esthetic implant restoration. Int J Periodontics Restorative Dent. 1997 Dec;17(6),584–91.

Jemt T. Regeneration of gingival papillae after single implant treatment. Int J Periodontics Restorative Dent. 1997 Aug; 17(4):326–33.

Jemt T. Restoring the gingival contour by means of provisional resin crowns after single-implant treatment. Int J Periodontics Restorative Dent. 1999 Feb;19(1):20–9.

Jung RE, Siegenthaler DW, Hämmerle CH. Postextraction tissue management: a soft tissue punch technique. Int J Periodontics Restorative Dent. 2004 Dec;24(6):545–53.

Kan JY, Rungcharassaeng K, Umezu K, Kois JC. Dimensions of peri-implant mucosa: An evaluation of maxillary anterior single implants in humans. J Periodontol. 2003 Apr;74(4):557–62.

Karroussis IK, Salvi GE, Heitz-Mayfield LJ, Bragger U, Hämmerle CH, Lang NP. Long-term implant prognosis in patients with and without a history of chronic periodontitis: a 10-year prospective cohort study of the ITI Dental Implant System. Clin Oral Implants Res. 2003 Jun;14(3):329–39.

Kohal RJ, Weng D. Bachle M, Strub JR. Loaded custom-made zirconia and titanium implants show similar osseointegration: an animal experiment. J Periodontol. 2004 Sep;75(9):1262–8.

Kois JC, Kan JY. Predictable peri-implant gingival aesthetics: Surgical and prosthodontic rationales. Pract Proced Aesthet Dent. 2001 Nov-Dec;13(9):691–8; quiz 700, 721–2.

Kornman KS, Crane A, Wang HY, di Giovine FS, Newman MG, Pirk FW, et al. The interleukin-1 genotype as a severity factor in adult periodontal disease. J Clin Periodontol. 1997 Jan;24(1):72–7.

Lambert PM, Morris HF, Ochi S. The influence of smoking on 3-year clinical success of osseointegrated dental implants. Ann Periodontol. 2000 Dec;5(1):79 – 89.

Landsberg CJ. Socket seal surgery combined with immediate implant placement: a novel approach for single-tooth replacement. Int J Periodontics Restorative Dent. 1997 Apr;17(2):140 – 9.

Lekholm U. Clinical procedures for treatment with osseointegrated dental implants. J Prosthet Dent. 1983 Jul;50(1):116 – 20.

Lindeboom JA, Tjiook Y, Kroon FH. Immediate placement of implants in periapical infected sites: a prospective randomized study in 50 patients. Oral Surg Oral Med Oral Pathol Oral Radiol Endod. 2006 Jun;101(6):705 – 10. Epub 2006 Mar 22.

Lüthy H, Pietrobon N, Sisera M, Wohlwend A, Loeffel O. White Esthetics. Schweiz Monatsschr Zahnmed. 1996;106 (10):896 – 908.

Markus SJ. Interim esthetic restorations in conjunction with anterior implants. J Prosthet Dent. 1999 Aug;82(2):233 – 36.

Morton D, Martin WC, Ruskin JD. Single-stage Straumann dental implants in the aesthetic zone: considerations and treatment procedures. J Oral Maxillofac Surg. 2004 Sep;62(9 Suppl 2):57 – 66.

Moskowitz EM, Sheridan JJ, Celenza F Jr, Tovilo K, Munoz AM. Essix appliances. Provisional anterior prosthesis for pre- and post-implant patients. N Y State Dent J. 1997 Apr;63(4):32 – 5.

Nieri M, Muzzi L, Cattabriga M, Rotundo R, Cairo F, Pini Prato GP. The prognostic value of several periodontal factors measured as radiographic bone level variation: a 10- year retrospective multilevel analysis of treated and maintained periodontal patients. J Periodontol. 2002 Dec;73(12):1485 – 93.

Oates TW, West J, Jones J, Kaiser D, Cochran DL. Long-term changes in soft tissue height on the facial surface of dental implants. Implant Dent. 2002;11(3):272 – 9.

Paul SJ, Jovanovic SA. Anterior implant-supported reconstructions: a prosthetic challenge. Pract Periodontics Aesthet Dent. 1999 Jun-Jul;11(5):585 – 90; quiz 592.

Potashnick SR. Soft tissue modeling for the esthetic single-tooth implant restoration. J Esthet Dent. 1998;10(3):121 – 31.

Priest G. Predictability of soft tissue form around single-tooth implant restorations. Int J Periodontics Restorative Dent. 2003 Feb;23(1):19 – 27.

Proceedings of the ITI Consensus Conference. Clin Oral Implants Res. 2000;11 Suppl 1:1 – 158.

Proceedings of the Third ITI Consensus Conference. Int J Oral Maxillofac Implants. 2004;19 Suppl:1 – 156.

Proffit WR, Fields HW. Contemporary Orthodontics. 2nd ed. St. Louis:Mosby Year Book; 1992

Saadoun AP, Sullivan DY, Krischek M, Le Gall M. Single tooth implant – management for success. Pract Periodontics Aesthet Dent. 1994 Apr;6(3):73 – 80; quiz 82.

Salama H, Salama M, Garber DA. Techniques for developing optimal peri-implant papillae within the esthetic zone. I. Guided soft tissue augmentation: The three-stage approach. J Esthet Dent. 1995;7(3):3 – 9.

Salama H, Salama M, Kelly J. The orthodontic-periodontal connection in implant site development. Pract Periodontics Aesthet Dent. 1996 Nov-Dec;8(9):923-32; quiz 934.

Seghi RR, Denry IL, Rosenstiel SF. Relative fracture toughness and hardness of new dental ceramics. J Prosthet Dent. 1995 Aug;74(2):145 – 50.

Shimpuku H, Nosaka Y, Kawamura T, Tachi Y, Shinohara M, Ohura K. Genetic polymorphisms of the interleukin-1 gene and early marginal bone loss around endosseous dental implants. Clin Oral Implants Res. 2003 Aug;14(4):423 – 9.

Small PN, Tarnow DP. Gingival recession around implants: a 1-year longitudinal prospective study. Int J Oral Maxillofac Implants. 2000 Jul-Aug;15(4):527 – 32.

Tai H, Endo M, Shimada Y, Gou E, Orima K, Kobayashi T, et al. Association of interleukin receptor antagonist gene polymorphisms with early onset periodontitis in Japanese. J Clin Periodontol. 2002 Oct;29(10):882 – 8.

Takei HH.The interdental space. Dent Clin North Am. 1980 Apr;24(2):169 – 76.

Tarnow DP, Magner AW, Fletcher P. The effect of the distance from the contact point to the crest of bone on the presence or absence of the interproximal dental papilla. J Periodontol. 1992 Dec;63(12):995 – 6.

Tarnow DP, Cho SC, Wallace SS. The effect of inter-implant distance on the height of inter-implant bone crest. J Periodontol. 2000 Apr;71(4):546 – 9.

Tarnow D, Elian N, Fletcher P, Froum S, Magner A, Cho SC, et al. Vertical distance from the crest of bone to the height of the interproximal papilla between adjacent implants. J Periodontol. 2003; Dec;74(12):1785-8.

Touati B. Improving aesthetics of implant-supported restorations. Pract Periodontics Aesthet Dent. 1995 Nov-Dec;7(9):81 – 92; quiz 93.

Vogel RC: Enhancing implant esthetics with ideal provisionalization. J Indiana Dent Assoc. 2002 Fall;81(3):11 – 4.

Wallace RH. The relationship between cigarette smoking and dental implant failure. Eur J Prosthodont Restor Dent. 2000 Sep;8(3):103 – 6.

Weisgold AS. Contours of the full crown restoration. Alpha Omegan. 1977 Dec;70(3):77 – 89.

Zitzmann NU, Naef R, Schärer P. Resorbable versus nonresorbable membranes in combination with Bio-Oss for guided bone regeneration. Int J Oral Maxillofac Implants. 1997 Jul-Aug;12(6):844 – 52.